AII IN THE FAMILY

Libby Spurrier lives in London with her husband and three children. She has had varied jobs in BBC radio, her primary career for all her working life, on programmes such as *The Long March of Everyman*, *Kaleidoscope*, *The Year in Question* and for ten years on *Bookshelf*. She currently works for *Woman's Hour*. This is her first book.

AIDS IN THE FAMILY

LIBBY SPURRIER

Hodder & Stoughton
LONDON SYDNEY AUCKLAND

The poem 'AIDS' is from *Halfway to Silence* by May Sarton,
first published by The Women's Press Ltd (1993),
34 Great Sutton Street, London EC1V 0DX,
and is used by permission of The Women's Press Ltd.

First published in Great Britain 1994

British Library Cataloguing in Publication Data

Spurrier, Libby
AIDS in the Family
I. Title
362.1969792

ISBN 0-340-58973-6

Photoset by Rowland Phototypesetting Ltd,
Bury St Edmunds, Suffolk

Printed and bound in Great Britain by
Mackays of Chatham plc, Chatham, Kent

Hodder and Stoughton Ltd
A Division of Hodder Headline PLC
47 Bedford Square
London WC1B 3DP

CONTENTS

FOREWORD

For several reasons I am particularly pleased to be asked to write a Foreword for this book, *Aids in the Family*. Its genesis is the experience of the author, Libby Spurrier, following the painful discovery that her brother Charles, also an old friend and colleague of mine, is living with AIDS. With refreshing honesty, Libby admits that researching and writing the book was her way of coming to terms with such a challenging turn of events, even though she had long suspected the truth.

With this personal experience as her starting point, Libby has interviewed the contributors with great sensitivity and skill. This has enabled them too to tell their stories honestly, and in the kind of detail which I am sure will help readers understand the issues, think for themselves and anticipate some of what may lie ahead.

Much has been written about HIV and AIDS, and from many angles. My shelves are stuffed with books on the subject; books by scientists, clinicians, nurses, social researchers, activisits and by people living with the virus. But so far there has been very little written about the impact of this virus on families.

This excellent book introduces the reader to the complicated and frightening world of HIV and AIDS with straightforward facts presented in a digestible form, as well as to some of the issues which are particular to families. It then draws, often very movingly, on Libby's interviews with mothers and fathers, brothers and sisters, lovers, husbands and wives of people who have lived with, and died of AIDS. This fills a significant gap in the bibliography.

What the years of working with this issue have taught me is that our own experience is the safest, perhaps the only place to start. The great strength of the response to the epidemic the world over is that so much of it is born of direct experience, and nourished by a courageous refusal to be victimised.

Aids in the Family does not fall into the trap of offering any formula. It states facts and shares the stories of others. Embracing the reality of AIDS, and coming to terms with its consequences, is a challenge every affected family will have to meet with its own particular, fresh response. I believe this book can be a great help, not least in reminding its readers that they are not alone.

Christopher Spence
Director
London Lighthouse

AUTHOR NOTE

One evening in January 1991 the phone rang. It was my sister-in-law, my younger brother's wife. I knew when she said "Have you got five minutes?" that it wasn't just a routine chat. The news she had for me was that she had that morning taken my other brother into St Mary's Paddington where he had been admitted with what the hospital suspected was PCP (Pneumocystis carinii pneumonia).

As the AIDS cases increased, my parents, my sister and my younger brother had all wondered whether he might have caught the virus. However, my husband and I had one great friend who was a haemophiliac and from what he told me about his HIV condition I had suspected that my brother had indeed become HIV positive.

It was a huge trauma visiting him in hospital that first time, seeing him so ill, drugged and wired-up with drips. After one or two setbacks, notably a horrible reaction to the drug he was being treated with which actually put him back in hospital, he recovered completely. He then enjoyed about a year and a half of moderately good health.

In June 1992 he rang me one evening at the weekend and said he felt very unwell and suspected he might have PCP again. We rang the ward at St Bartholomew's Hospital in London where his medical team, under Professor Tony Pinching, had moved from St Mary's. They said the best thing would be to bring him in and they'd start doing some X-rays in order to reach a diagnosis.

It did turn out to be PCP and he was in hospital for about three weeks. Then he came home to convalesce with me and my family. After about a week he began to feel very ill again. He tried to walk to the post box at the end of the road, and barely managed to stagger home again. So at the end of that first week I took him back into hospital. I remember it vividly – I had to take my younger son and one of his friends with me as they were having a day off school and I felt terribly guilty about dragging them into a hospital in the middle of London on a boiling hot June day.

My brother then spent another three weeks in hospital, looking, if possible, even iller than before. It was during that second stay that I had the idea for this book.

I had arrived to visit my brother as his doctor was coming to see him. The doctor was extremely helpful and told us exactly what he was doing and what drugs he was using. What he actually said was that he didn't know exactly what was wrong with my brother – it could be the PCP again, or it could be TB. Whatever it was, he was too ill for them to wait for the results of the various tests to get a diagnosis before beginning treatment.

So what the doctor was doing was treating all the things he suspected my brother might have with a sophisticated cocktail of drugs – "treating presumptively" was how he put it. It became quite clear to me during our conversation that there was no point in asking the doctor for a prognosis of what might happen. How could he know? All he could do was treat whatever he could with every drug he had.

I felt I would be much better prepared for what might happen in our family if I had some idea of what other people had gone through. But, as a working mother of three I felt I had neither the time nor perhaps the inclination to go and join a support group, or seek out counselling. The books I found in the library were either complicated and frightening textbooks, or stories about people who were themselves HIV positive but not actually ill. I read most of them, and learned a lot.

I remember when I was about to have my first child, fourteen years ago, I read a paperback which just had women's stories of their childbirth experiences. I was absolutely riveted by their stories, as I now might be by mothers' accounts of dealings with teenagers!

For this book I have talked to fathers and mothers, sisters and brothers, lovers and wives and friends of people with AIDS. I didn't find it easy, not least because I found their stories almost unbearably moving to listen to. They have all coped with the most amazing trials and tribulations with an enormous amount of courage. Above all they have without exception been terribly kind and supportive to me.

I have been fascinated by their accounts as I've worked on them, partly because every story turned out to be different and I didn't plan it that way! In a way it was like gathering together a support group – I learnt a lot, but I was also very glad to find so many experiences common to us all. The main example of this is the difficulty of adjusting between crisis illnesses in a relative with AIDS and the periods in between of good health. Time and time again families have said they have found this one of the most tiring and emotionally draining factors.

I hope their stories will help other families and friends in similar positions. I would have liked to have included more interviews with women who have AIDS, particularly to underline that AIDS is not confined to any one group; that they are under-represented in the accounts that follow is not from want of trying.

I am enormously grateful to all those who allowed me to use their stories in this book. I thank them too for their enthusiasm and encouragement of the project – and above all for their friendship.

I owe a special debt to Sister Eva Heymann, who knows everybody, and who has allowed me to take up hours of her time. She has been wonderfully supportive and I couldn't have done it without her.

I would also like to thank my brother, Charles Maude, for his support and for his expert advice.

I have sometimes referred to the person with AIDS as he for the sake of simplicity although many women are affected by the virus.

Libby Spurrier
August 1993

GLOSSARY

ACYCLOVIR
Drug used to treat herpes.

AIDS
Acquired Immune Deficiency Syndrome. The condition where the immune system is weakened, leaving the body unable to resist certain infections and cancers which may be serious and in some cases fatal. Syndrome because it is a collection of symptoms and illnesses. Someone cannot be said to have AIDS until they have suffered from one or more of the symptoms.

ALTERNATIVE THERAPIES
Treatments outside conventional medicine, sometimes available on the National Health Service. These include homeopathy, aromatherapy massage, acupuncture, chiropractic and herbal medicine. Many of these treatments concentrate on the treatment of the whole body rather than specific symptoms. Names and addresses can be found through Holistic Medicine organisations or through places such as the South London Natural Health Centre in Clapham. Treatments usually cost around £25 a time.

AIDS RELATED COMPLEX (ARC)
A minor deficiency in the immune system which results from HIV infection. Symptoms includes fevers, oral thrush, night sweats and weight loss. Although disabling, these symptoms do not add up to AIDS and do not qualify people for the full range of benefits and social services available to those with an "official" diagnosis of AIDS. A term rarely used these days.

AZT

Azidothymidine or Zidovudine, marketed as Retrovir. One of the few anti-retroviral drugs licensed in Britain, i.e. it is used to fight the HIV virus. It's taken in tablet form and many people with HIV take it in lower dosages than those originally recommended. It supposedly works by helping to block the virus's replication inside the infected cell and so prevent the development of full-blown AIDS. It was originally developed to fight cancer but was withdrawn because of the toxic side effects, which include anaemia, headaches, nausea, damage to the bone marrow and muscle wasting. In March 1993 the Medical Research Council announced that the drug has now been proved not to have been effective in preventing the onset of AIDS in people with HIV. It is still prescribed to people with AIDS and is believed to be useful combined with other anti-retroviral drugs.

BRONCHOSCOPY

A procedure used to establish the cause of infection in the lungs. A thin instrument is pushed down the throat into the lungs to remove samples for tests. Usually carried out under mild sedation.

CANDIDA ALBICANS

A common fungus present in most humans, causing thrush, but usually controlled by the immune system. The most common cause of mouth problems in HIV illness. It causes inflammation and soreness in the mouth and can spread into the oesophagus. Common treatment is with Fluconazole.

CMV – CYTOMEGALOVIRUS

A virus of the herpes group, transmitted through body fluids, which is carried by large numbers of the general population. In people with HIV it can affect the nervous system, the intestines, and sometimes the lungs. The most serious effect however is on the eyes – it can cause blindness. Treatment includes Gancyiclovir and Foscarnet.

DAPSONE

A drug used to treat and prevent AIDS-related pneumonia.

DDI – DIDEOXYINOSINE

A more recently developed anti-HIV drug than AZT. An anti-retroviral drug, i.e. it is used to fight the HIV virus, which is closely related to but less toxic than AZT and does not cause bone marrow damage. However, the side effects can include inflammation of the pancreas, abdominal pain and fever. Like AZT, it does not offer a cure and does not prevent the onset of full-blown AIDS.

DDU

A drug dependency unit.

DEMENTIA

Loss of memory, difficulty with writing and reading, and disorientation caused by the direct effect of the HIV virus on the brain.

FACTOR 8

Protein in the blood which is necessary for the formation of blood clots. Factor 8 is not present in the blood of haemophiliacs.

FAIDS

Feline AIDS. Caused by a similar retrovirus to that which causes feline leukaemia. It damages the cat's immune system, leaving the cat vulnerable to illnesses such as chest infections and pneumonia. Humans cannot catch HIV or AIDS from cats, but cats do catch it from each other through saliva. Now quite common in the cat population, especially in some areas of London.

FANSIDAR

The drug used to prevent the occurrence of AIDS-related pneumonia.

FLUCONAZOLE

The drug to treat candida albicans.

GP

General practitioner or family doctor.

GU
Genito urinary clinic or ward.

HAEMOPHILIA
A genetically inherited condition affecting mainly men, in which the blood lacks the protein called Factor 8 which clots the blood. Haemophiliacs require regular quantities of Factor 8 which is given in blood transfusions. Before 1985 unscreened blood was used which was later found to contain HIV, thus infecting many haemophiliacs.

HERPES SIMPLEX
The virus that causes cold sores and ulcers on the genitals. Treated with Acyclovir.

HIV
Human Immunodeficiency Virus. A slow-acting virus which attacks the "helper" cells in the blood system, i.e. the cells which alert the immune system to fight off infections. The immune system of the person affected is damaged and weakened, leaving the body open to infections which may cause a variety of illnesses.

HIV ENCEPHALOPATHY
A neurological disease which shows as memory loss, confusion, personality changes, and may progress to dementia and incontinence. The drug Zidovudine has in the past been used to try to delay or prevent onset.

HIV POSITIVE
Someone who is infected with the HIV virus.

KS – KAPOSI'S SARCOMA
Purplish skin tumour which many people with AIDS develop. It was first noticed long before AIDS in men over sixty from the Mediterranean. Kaposi's Sarcoma appears on the skin as purple patches. It is much more common in homosexual patients and is usually benign. Kaposi's Sarcoma also affects the lungs, intestines

and lymph nodes. Radio and chemotherapy is often offered as treatment.

THE LONDON LIGHTHOUSE
A centre for people with HIV and AIDS situated in west London. It provides hospice and respite care, advice and support. Open since 1988. Address on page 216.

MAI
Mycobacterium Avium Intracellulare. A form of TB, rarer than ordinary TB, which causes lung problems and diarrhoea. MAI is slow to respond to antibiotics, but can be treated with Rifabutin or Ethambutol. Treatment can be long-term.

MENINGITIS, CRYPTOCOCCAL
An infection of the brain tissue caused by the yeast bacteria Cryptococcus neoformans.

MILDMAY MISSION HOSPITAL
One of the few hospices for people with AIDS, situated in the East End of London. Address on page 217.

NEBULISER
A device for spraying drugs in aerosol form into the lungs. Used originally in asthma, now used for pentamidine prophylaxis for PCP.

PCP
Pneumocystis carinii pneumonia, a form of pneumonia which is AIDS-related and quite difficult to diagnose – a bronchoscopy is usually performed whereby an instrument is pushed down into the lungs to remove samples for tests. In days before prophylaxis most people with AIDS outside Africa would experience PCP at some stage in the illness. Very often this is the first illness which attacks someone with HIV. It responds well to antibiotics, usually Septrin or Pentamidine, which is administered in hospital intravenously, i.e. with a drip. Both drugs have side effects, most notably of skin rashes and nausea, although new drugs are being designed all the

17

time which help to counteract these. Treatment usually means two or three weeks in hospital before several weeks or months of convalescence. Drugs may well then have to be taken by the patient prophylactically, that is, to be taken in tablet form every day, in order to prevent a further occurrence of PCP. Many people with AIDS take the drug pentamidine through a nebuliser at home every couple of weeks to protect against infection.

PENTAMIDINE
One of the most effective drugs used to treat AIDS-related pneumonia, given intravenously while in hospital and also in tablet form or through a nebuliser at prescribed intervals.

PGL
Persistent Generalised Lymphadenopathy.

PROPHYLAXIS
Treatment usually with drugs or homeopathic medicine which is designed to be taken when well to prevent illnesses occurring.

REHAB
Abbreviation for drug rehabilitation unit where drug addicts go to undergo supervised detoxification.

SAIDS
SIMIAN AIDS, or AIDS in monkeys. How close simian versions are to the human immunodeficiency virus is controversial and is at the heart of the debate about where AIDS originated.

SALMONELLA
Food poisoning. Dangerous for those with HIV as it may get into the blood stream and cause severe illness. When cooking for someone with HIV it is very important to observe good food hygiene.

SEPTRIN
Drug used to treat AIDS-related pneumonia. Given intravenously and in tablet form.

SHINGLES

A painful and itchy rash which follows infection by the herpes zoster virus, the same virus which causes chickenpox in children. An adult with HIV who has never had chickenpox should avoid contact with a child with chickenpox, which can be fatal to someone with AIDS. People with shingles should avoid contact with someone with AIDS.

STD

Sexually transmissable disease. Any disease which is caught through sexual activity, such as herpes, syphilis and Hepatitis B.

T-CELL, also T4 cells, CD4, or Helper cells

White cells in the blood. These form a crucial part of the cellular immune system. Their job is to help the response of the immune system in fighting infection. If the "T-Cell count" is lower than average, the immune system is weakened.

TERRENCE HIGGINS TRUST

Set up in 1983 in London in memory of Terrence Higgins, one of the first people to die of AIDS in Britain. It provides support, information and advice to people affected by HIV and AIDS. Address on page 218.

TOXOPLASMOSIS

An illness caused by a micro-organism called TOXOPLASMA GONDII which lives in the intestines of cats. Toxoplasmosis can affect babies in the womb causing blindness and brain damage. In people with HIV, toxoplasmosis mainly affects the brain, causing abscesses which in turn lead to severe headaches, loss of co-ordination, and possibly loss of movement on one side of the body. Toxoplasmosis is caused by a protozoon and it responds well to treatment with drugs such as Septrin, Dapsone, Clindamycin and Fansidar.

VIRUS

One of the simplest of all living organisms, which land on living cells and attach themselves like a parasite.

WORKS

A term used by intravenous drug users to describe injecting equipment, such as needles, syringes, spoons and filters.

1
Practicalities

The fear of AIDS affects us all. If you don't know someone who has been diagnosed HIV positive, you will probably have read the newspapers over the last few years and become aware of the growing number of famous people who have been lost through AIDS in this country and abroad. Indeed it would have been hard not to notice the passing of the ballet dancer Rudolph Nureyev or the wonderful English actor Denholm Elliott, the much-loved pop star Freddie Mercury and the tennis player Arthur Ashe. There has also been a fair amount of publicity about people living with AIDS, like the film director Derek Jarman and the basketball player Magic Johnson.

In America most people know someone with AIDS or someone who has been bereaved because of the illness. In the developed West and in the United States the disease is still proportionately higher in the homosexual community than amongst heterosexuals. However, the rate of HIV diagnosis is now rising faster among women and children than among gay men, and fastest among young heterosexuals. This means that we are all likely to come into contact with AIDS sooner or later – a friend will lose a brother, a mother a son and daughter-in-law, a wife will lose a husband and perhaps know that she will eventually die too.

When we're frightened, it's difficult to think about the implications of illness, let alone talk about them. It used to be the same with cancer and mental illness. Nobody wanted to discuss cancer openly – it was just not something you told the neighbours about if it occurred in your family, and mental illness was something to be ashamed of. Now mental illnesses have been given different labels such as Alzheimers and schizophrenia and are more easily understood, cancer is respectable and often curable, and we have AIDS, a terrifying and powerful new virus.

Many people in this country still know very little about related HIV illness, and that means that there is a great deal of fear and prejudice around. When a person becomes infected with HIV, his or her family and friends are in turn affected – the family in particular may feel frightened that they will be shunned by friends and may not know where to turn to for help and advice. So at the very time in our lives when we may be facing a crisis with a likely bereavement – when we need our friends and neighbours, our family doctor, our parish priest and our school teachers to know what we're going through, to give us as much support as possible – families often don't find the support they need.

In the mid-1980s the advertising campaigns run by the British Government to educate people about HIV used some terrifying images, not least that of the huge gravestone falling over. To those who didn't know much about AIDS and who thought it would never happen to them, these advertisements seem to have reinforced fear and prejudice and hindered understanding.

At the same time the forecasts predicting an AIDS epidemic in Britain were quoting figures of up to 40,000 people who would have AIDS by the end of 1992. This in itself has added to our fear even though these figures have not been realised. Although the images in the advertisements seem to have raised levels both of awareness and anxiety about HIV, the campaign itself, which stressed the need to practise safer sex in order to stop the virus from spreading, does not seem to have changed people's sexual behaviour.

In her introduction to her book *Terminal Care for People with AIDS* Dr Veronica Moss, Medical Director of the Mildmay Mission Hospital in London, states that young heterosexual people on the whole have not accepted the need for a change in attitude towards casual sex. In other words, the feeling that "it won't happen to me" is still common. Even by October 1987 in the United States, the rate of newly detected HIV infection was twice as high amongst heterosexuals as among homosexuals and bisexuals. In the United Kingdom the number of HIV infected heterosexual men and women almost doubled during 1990[1] and still continues to rise.

However, in Britain, unlike the Third World, homosexual and

[1] THTHAB and CDSC.

bisexual men make up 80 per cent of all AIDS cases and 66 per cent of HIV infected people who have been tested.

The statistics compiled by the Communicable Diseases Surveillance Centre[2] reveal that since the figures began to be reported in 1982, a total of 7,699 cases of AIDS have been reported in Britain. Of this figure, 7,140 are male and 559 female. The number of deaths from AIDS as at June 1993 was 4,794. The number of people reported with HIV was 19,989 in June 1993. Of this number, 60 per cent were exposed to HIV through sexual intercourse between men; 13 per cent through sexual intercourse between men and women; 12 per cent through intravenous drug use, and 1 per cent through intravenous drug use combined with sexual intercourse between men. By the end of June 1993, a total of 118 AIDS cases in children under the age of 14 was reported, in addition to 451 cases of children with HIV. Clearly this figure cannot include those people who are unaware they have caught the virus.

In 99.99 per cent of cases throughout the world, HIV is transmitted through unsafe sex, sharing contaminated needles, or through contaminated blood products.[3]

By January 1991 there was some evidence that there were members of the gay community who were rejecting the message of safer sex which is put across so strongly by organisations like the Terrence Higgins Trust. It seemed that gay men under the age of twenty-five had decided it was quite safe to have unprotected sex with each other, in the belief that only men in their thirties and forties develop AIDS.[4]

The rise in HIV infection among heterosexuals also suggests that the message of safer sex isn't getting across, or that sex education is failing to reach those who are most at risk from infection.

By the year 2000, there may be a global total of 15 to 20 million adults, and 10 million children with AIDS. By 1993 the number of people infected with HIV worldwide was 14 million, of which a large proportion was found in Africa.

[2] CDSC.
[3] NAM.
[4] Judy Tavanyar, Terrence Higgins Trust *HIV/AIDS Book*, Thorsons.

On World AIDS Day 1990, Dr Michael Merson, the Director of the WHO's Global AIDS Programme, said that an estimated 1 in 40 African women, 1 in 500 South American women and 1 in 700 North American women were infected with the virus – a global total of around 3 million.

Dr Lorraine Sherr[5] says that by the end of the century up to 500,000 children will have lost one or both parents from AIDS; 10 per cent of those under 15 in 10 African countries will be AIDS orphans; and in New York between 50,000 and 100,000 children will lose one parent to AIDS.

Emotionally we have moved on since the early 1980s, when there was such ignorance about the virus that it was regarded with almost hysterical fear: in one part of Britain parents refused to send their children to school with a haemophiliac boy who was HIV positive and telephone engineers refused to do repairs to the Gay Switchboard telephones in London for fear of "catching AIDS" from the telephones. Elsewhere, a group of Oxford dons (presumably a moderately intelligent bunch of men) decided to stop an ancient tradition of passing a "loving cup" of wine around the dinner table in case the virus could be caught through saliva, and there have been lots of questions asked about drinking from the chalice in church at the communion rail.

Although there is less hysteria about HIV and AIDS there is still a surprising lack of knowledge about the virus, how it is contracted and when full-blown AIDS occurs.

FAMILIES

Families may not want to know too much about the illness, but if they do want information they need it as quickly as possible. The time they will need help most is usually when they find out about the diagnosis in a relative.

[5] Dr Lorraine Sherr, *HIV and AIDS in Mothers and Babies*, Blackwell Scientific Publications.

If the person with HIV has taken the family into his confidence from the beginning, then there may be several years before anything goes wrong and the family will have space in which to absorb the implications and learn a bit about what the future may bring, if that's what they want.

But when the knowledge of the diagnosis only comes with the first illness there will seem to be very little time to get informed. It is likely too that the person with AIDS will be incredibly well informed. They may well have been reading about the syndrome for the several years since they were diagnosed with HIV and before getting ill. So easy-to-understand information is vital. In that respect I hope this book will help.

There are two main differences which families of people with AIDS encounter which separate them from families who are having to cope with cancer or other terminal illnesses.

The first main difference for families with AIDS is that because it is a syndrome, not an illness in itself, there will be many different illnesses which will affect the person with AIDS. Nobody will ever be able to tell you what illness might come next.

One of the striking things about people with AIDS is their ability to deal with and fight illness after illness. There are people who have had PCP, and recovered completely; meningitis, and recovered; salmonella, and recovered; toxoplasmosis, and recovered; let alone managing to live extremely well with lingering forms of TB.

The sheer determination of people with AIDS to get better and leave hospital is amazing. I remember going into an AIDS ward in a London hospital and seeing a woman who didn't look as if she could possibly last the night, and did indeed have what seemed like all her family and friends keeping vigil in her room. Two days later she was sitting on her bed, dressed in a track suit, smoking a fag, waiting for her family to take her home, chirpy as anything.

A person with AIDS may have to suffer many potentially terminal illnesses, such as *PCP* or *toxoplasmosis, meningitis*, or *salmonella*. But as drugs become more sophisticated and effective with every day that passes, so the outlook for AIDS patients improves all the time. For instance, some of the people in this book became ill in the 1980s and there was very little treatment

27

then for PCP or for CMV (cytomegalovirus). Today both illnesses are treatable and respond extremely well to anti-biotics.

Each serious illness will require hospitalisation probably for several weeks. Each illness is an anxious and extremely stressful time for family and friends. Hospital visiting is very exhausting, especially if the visitors have to travel long distances to London. Your friend or relative may be well for months and years at a time, and may never have more than one identifiable illness.

He or she may have all the possible permutations of all the various illnesses. No one can predict what may happen.

It is sometimes hard for doctors to be certain when someone has entered a terminal stage of the illness. Friends and family may find that having tried to prepare themselves for the worst, the patient recovers completely and will go on to enjoy a long spell of good health and may have years of good quality life left. One mother told me one of the most difficult things about the AIDS illnesses was simply the fact it goes on for such a long time but is punctuated with dramas. Every time her son goes into hospital she drops everything and devotes herself to being with him, only to find two weeks later he's better, coping well again at home, and she has to pick up her life again until the next time.

This makes life stressful. Dr Lorraine Sherr, a psychologist at St Mary's Hospital, Paddington, described it to me as "not knowing what gear to be in". A family may spend a week or two of intense anxiety in a crisis situation while the person with AIDS lies seriously ill in hospital. Parents, siblings and friends may feel they have to visit every day, there may be lots of extra work in terms of washing and shopping, and it may well be a very time-consuming and exhausting period. That of course is true for anyone having relatives and friends in hospital.

Then there comes the convalescence, and the time when the person with AIDS feels well enough to resume his or her life and enjoy some good quality living on his or her own territory, if that is possible. This is the chance for everyone to stand back and relax, but it is difficult not to go on feeling anxious about the patient. The sister of a man with AIDS I interviewed described this as "walking the tightrope". I know that after my brother has been ill in hospital and convalesced with us for a month before he feels

28

well enough to go back to his own flat, it takes me a week to get myself back to normal, to where my own family was before he got ill.

However, it may be years before the next crisis occurs. Some families who have been through many such crises occasionally surprise nursing staff who have not met them before by their laid-back approach. Some families and friends don't visit as much during the second illness as during the first, and less and less as the illnesses progress. They may have reacted with such intensity during previous hospitalisations that they may have temporarily exhausted their emotional ability even to grieve.

There is no doubt that a succession of potentially fatal illnesses does mean that family members and friends will find themselves facing bereavement several times, and grieving in advance of the actual death of the person.

Secondly, families of people with AIDS may have to deal with the undoubted stigma which is attached to the illness. It is necessary to be quite honest about this and recognise that this is because in the majority of AIDS cases, the virus has been caught through sex. In general, British people don't talk about sex within the family circle, although we may talk to friends and partners about it. On the whole sex is something we are embarrassed about and it is this which makes many families fearful to tell their own friends and neighbours what is wrong with their son or daughter. We worry about what the neighbours will think.

This book has been written to try to provide information about how AIDS occurs, and to show through the various stories what may happen during the course of the illness. Every story turns out to be slightly different, which serves to illustrate the point that one never knows what to expect next. It also aims to give practical information which will help the reader to seek help and resources when they need them, and how to cope emotionally as well as practically.

WHAT IS AIDS?

AIDS stands for Acquired Immune Deficiency Syndrome. It means that the body's immune system has been damaged so that it can no longer fight off infection. It is generally accepted that AIDS develops in a person who has caught HIV (Human Immunodeficiency Virus). * The virus enters the blood stream and attacks the "helper" cells in the blood. Once these cells are damaged by the virus, the immune system isn't strong enough to fight off infections that normal healthy bodies resist without the owner of that body even being aware of it. The defence system which keeps people healthy becomes gradually weaker. For instance a healthy person may not catch the TB virus or the common viral pneumonias that are floating around in the air, but people with a damaged immune system are far more likely to. It is usually these illnesses, not the virus itself, which weakens the person and causes them to become seriously ill and sometimes to die.

Being diagnosed as HIV positive does not however mean instant or even inevitable illness. Because HIV is a very slow-acting virus it is usually several years before the infected person shows any sign of ill health. Sometimes they don't become ill at all and continue with their life unaware that they have been infected with the virus.

However, a person who is HIV positive can develop several illnesses before AIDS develops. These include PGL (Persistent Generalised Lymphadenopathy) and ARC (AIDS related complex) which while debilitating are not life-threatening.

A person develops AIDS when he or she becomes ill with one of several serious illnesses. It may be that a person with HIV begins to feel very unwell and breathless, and this may turn out to be PCP, a life-threatening illness which is quite often the first serious illness people with HIV experience. In fact almost half of AIDS cases have PCP when they are initially diagnosed.

---

* Although some scientists dispute this, only adding to the debate about how AIDS is contracted.

HOW THE HIV VIRUS IS CONTRACTED

Research has shown that the HIV virus can be present in the blood, breastmilk, urine, faeces, semen, saliva, vaginal secretions, or rectal secretions of a person with HIV.

But the only body fluids which contain the virus in any quantity and therefore can pass on the virus are infected blood, semen and vaginal secretions and breastmilk.

At the time that someone becomes infected with the HIV virus himself, he may feel symptoms similar to flu for a couple of weeks. But after that when he feels better he may not be aware for years that he is HIV positive. During that time he may pass on the virus to anyone with whom he has unsafe sex, without him or his partners being aware of it.

HIV can be caught by having unprotected (that is without a condom) penetrative sex with someone who is already infected with HIV, even if that person is unaware that he or she has the virus.

Homosexual sex appears to carry a higher risk than sex between men and women, because the vagina is much tougher and less likely to suffer skin damage such as cuts and bruises than the anus. It seems possible that it is easier for the "passive" partner to catch the infection from the "active" partner than the other way round, but it would be very unsafe indeed to assume this. Studies suggest that the chance of a woman catching HIV during regular unprotected sex with an infected man is about one in four, compared to a one in ten chance for a man in the same relationship.[6] It also seems possible that a person in poor health, or someone whose immune system is depressed, may be more easily infected than a healthy and happy person.[7]

But everyone who has unprotected sex outside a monogamous relationship is at risk. Every new partner is a potential danger. It can take only one act of sexual intercourse to pass on or catch the virus. Every husband or wife who is unfaithful to their partner, particularly in countries where AIDS is more prevalent, puts not only themselves but their partner and any as yet unborn children at risk.

[6] Terrence Higgins Trust, *HIV AIDS Book*.
[7] *Understanding AIDS*, Dr John Starkie and Rodney Dale, Hodder & Stoughton.

You can be infected with the virus through a blood transfusion when the blood that is used has not been screened.

In Britain, except in Scotland, blood used to give transfusions to haemophiliacs, or anyone else, before 1985 was not screened for any infection at all, let alone HIV. However, since then, all blood is tested in this country. Blood always was screened in Scotland, so Scottish haemophiliacs were a great deal luckier than haemophiliacs in England and Wales.

In Britain every blood donor signs a form which gives permission for their blood to be screened for Hepatitis B and HIV. If a donor gives blood without knowing he is HIV positive, the blood transfusion centre will contact him and invite him back for counselling. They will then inform him of the result, and pass him back to his GP for treatment. They stress that they do not look after those people, but make every effort to trace them if their blood is HIV infected.

Blood donors are also asked to fill in a confidential questionnaire to establish whether they may be in a high-risk category. If there is any doubt at all about a person's status, they are advised not to donate blood. All needles used for taking blood in this country are used only once and then thrown away.

However, it can be dangerous to receive blood products, for example a transfusion after an accident, in foreign countries where blood is not screened for HIV antibodies. It is wise to discuss with your GP or the International Relations branch of the DSS before travelling abroad which countries screen blood and which do not. In poorer countries, the risk of contaminated equipment such as needles will also be higher. If travelling and in doubt, take a pack of new needles with you (these can be obtained at large chemists, through your GP or at major travel centres). As a general rule, in higher risk countries try to avoid treatment which involves injections and surgery, or blood from local blood donors.

You can catch the virus by injecting drugs into the bloodstream with a needle which has been used previously by someone else who is infected with the HIV virus, even though that person may not know he or she is already infected. This is because if a needle is shared, a small quantity of infected blood from the first person to inject can be injected into the second person's body along with the drug.

This is a particularly effective way to transmit HIV, as well as other infections such as septicaemia and Hepatitis B. The rules are always to use new or sterilised equipment. Injecting drug users can get clean needles from the needle exchange schemes which now exist in many areas. There are also new kinds of drug agencies which provide free, safe and anonymous help and advice (see pages 215–8).

By late 1986 the Scottish Committee on HIV said that about 50 per cent of injecting drug users in Scotland were infected with HIV.

People have caught the virus through having a tattoo done with infected needles. If you decide to have a tattoo always check that needles have not been used before. Similarly having your ears or nose pierced may be risky if the needles are shared or unsterilised. Most places that carry out ear piercing now use sophisticated and safe equipment in which a needle is used once and then thrown away. Unqualified people practising acupuncture or electrolysis might also be a risk. A careless practitioner might pass on contaminated blood from other clients. Always check that equipment is dealt with properly in terms of being sterilised, and if you're in doubt, go elsewhere.

A mother with HIV can pass the virus on to her baby in the womb, since HIV can cross the placenta. A baby might also be infected at birth through contact with infected vaginal fluid, though this is less likely. It is estimated that the chance that the virus can be passed on through infected breastmilk is around 30 per cent, so the advice to mothers who are HIV positive is to bottlefeed rather than breastfeed. Not all mothers with HIV will pass it on to the baby though, and babies cannot be tested for the virus at birth because all babies born to HIV positive mothers will still have their mother's antibodies. An HIV test at birth will detect the mother's antibodies to HIV that are still in the baby's bloodstream, even though the baby may not have inherited the virus. Testing for HIV infection is therefore not done until the baby is around 18 months old. Sadly, most babies who develop HIV will die from AIDS-related illnesses.

Not all pregnant women are offered the HIV test, although the Department of Health has said that it would like all pregnant women to be offered an HIV test routinely. Some hospitals do offer the test but in those hospitals such as the West London Hospital and St Bartholomew's in London, where the test has been offered since 1988, 6 out of 10 women take it up at St Bartholomew's and only 2 out of 10 at the West London.

For people wishing to be tested for HIV, the sensible thing is to go to a clinic. The majority of testing takes place in the STD or GUM clinics. There is usually such a clinic in most NHS hospitals.

The test is free, and anonymous, and you don't need an appointment. If you ask your GP to refer you for a test, that information may go on to your medical records, whatever the result of the test is, and may conceivably turn up in future years when you're trying to get a mortgage, life insurance or a new job.

Insurance companies almost always ask GPs if they can see confidential medical information about people asking for life and health insurance. Nowadays, life insurance companies insist they will not refuse a person life insurance because they have had an HIV test which proved negative, and have indeed given an assurance to the Government to this effect. They also state that if a test was taken as part of ante-natal screening, or at the request of another insurance company, it will be disregarded. However, if you take a test on your own initiative, they may use this as an indication of your lifestyle.[8]

Counselling is always given at the clinic, before and after you have the test and when you receive the result, which will be about ten days later. If you attend an STD clinic of your own accord, the results of the rest will remain there, although some clinics may want to inform your GP of the result. Alternatively you can visit a private clinic around Harley Street (for which you must pay) and you'll get the results the same day.

[8] NAM.

HOW YOU CANNOT CONTRACT HIV

Much of the fear surrounding HIV and AIDS has grown up because of the myths that you can catch the virus easily from someone who is HIV positive. This is nonsense. HIV is far less infectious than Hepatitis B, which is more often fatal.

You cannot catch the virus by breathing in the same air as someone who is HIV positive.

Although there have been small amounts of the virus found in saliva, it is in tiny amounts and not strong enough to cause infection. To put yourself at risk, you would have to inject yourself with about one pint of infected saliva.

So you cannot catch the virus by kissing someone, sharing a toothbrush, hugging someone, or shaking their hand. You cannot catch it by sharing a coffee cup. You cannot catch it from lavatory seats, or through sharing baths or showers.

You cannot catch it from sitting on the same chair as someone who is HIV positive.

You cannot catch AIDS from the swimming pool. The water in the pool dilutes the body fluids, and the chlorine kills the virus.

The virus lives only in body fluids. Although it's a devastating virus, it is a rather weak one.

It cannot live outside the body fluid for more than ten minutes. It does not survive in the acidity of the stomach contents, so you cannot catch it from vomit although if it has blood in it there is a slight risk.

No biting insect can transmit HIV infection, because of the tiny amount of blood they deal with. A sizeable quantity of blood needs to be passed for infection to occur, and the traces which have been found on insect's biting parts are not sufficient to cause infection. Bedbugs could in theory transmit the virus, but laboratory experiments have been conducted in which HIV is found only to survive for a very short time in the bedbug, and the tiny amount even a large tropical bedbug could pass from one person to another is far too little to be infectious.

You cannot catch it from mosquito bites, unless a thousand mosquitoes were fully trained to work like an army (which I suppose might just conceivably be believable in a James Bond film). And then they would have to bite someone infected with HIV, and then bite you within a few seconds.

There is no correlation between people who get bitten by mosquitoes and people who develop HIV infection, even among children who usually get bitten more.[9]

There have been cases in Britain of health care professionals such as doctors and midwives who have died from AIDS and there has been enormous public concern about the possible risks to patients who were looked after by them.

Doctors, nurses, dentists and other health professionals are not routinely tested for HIV. But all health care workers should routinely take steps to protect themselves from infection, for example, always wearing rubber gloves.

That in turn protects the patient. The BMA has issued general guidelines about the risk of infection, and points out that to date (1993) there have been no cases of HIV transmission from health care worker to patient, although there have been a few cases of staff catching the virus from a person with HIV, through needle stick injuries. (The risk of this happening is very low indeed.)

The Department of Health issued new and stringent guidelines to health care professionals in April 1993 and they stress that there have been no cases in this country of doctors or any other health care worker passing on the HIV virus to a patient.

The guidelines to local Health Authorities state that if a doctor or health care worker thinks he or she might be at risk of having caught HIV, he should be tested for the virus. This will be done in strict confidence. The names of those tested will not be released, and once the result is known there will be counselling about whether or not to change jobs. If the test is positive, in the case of a surgeon, this may mean stopping work at once, but in the case of a GP there would be no reason why he or she should cease practising. The Department of Health has also announced that a health care worker found to be HIV positive will be guaranteed a job somewhere within the Health Service.

GPs follow strict professional guidelines to protect both you and themselves, not just from HIV but from other diseases more

[9] Ibid.

infectious than HIV. Every instrument is sterilised, every needle thrown away after one use, and doctors wash thoroughly and wear rubber gloves.

The British Dental Association has issued a leaflet of guidelines which states "You won't catch AIDS through dental treatment", and they have also published guidelines on safe sterilisation and surgery hygiene procedures. Dentists must by law sterilise equipment between patients. These standard precautions are designed to protect dentist and patient. In the United States dental patients have been known to become HIV positive through unsterilised dental equipment.

Each District Health Authority has a duty to provide adequate dental treatment for people with AIDS, but individual contracts between dentists and the NHS give dentists the option to refuse treatment without giving a reason. If this happens to your relative, contact the District Dental Officer or your District Health Authority for advice. Dental treatment is usually available in hospitals.

HOW TO DEAL WITH HIV IN YOUR FAMILY

Some parents may not be fully aware of their child's lifestyle before their son or daughter becomes ill. Sometimes parents may not have faced up to the fact that their daughter has taken drugs or their son is gay, and may be genuinely unaware of the possibility. On an emotional level, it can be very difficult for parents of gay men to come to terms with the situation that not only is their son homosexual, but now he may be dying too. It may be even harder for a wife to lose her husband to AIDS and discover that she is HIV positive.

This is a lot to take on board all at once, and those involved will desperately need someone to talk to about how to cope. In most family situations there are usually some people who are excluded from the knowledge that a relative is HIV positive, perhaps because other family members feel they won't be able to cope and are protecting them. Each family has to decide for itself whom they will share the situation with. If the wider family, grand-mothers, aunts and cousins, are not included in the knowledge,

37

then that in itself can be a strain on the family members who do know. One friend of mine who became HIV through a blood transfusion would not tell his parents until shortly before he died, putting his wife and his brother, who did know, under a huge amount of stress.

I have heard people say "Oh, well AIDS is self induced isn't it?" The knowledge that this attitude exists makes it doubly hard for relatives and friends of someone with HIV to discuss and share their fears openly.

If there is fear and ignorance in the community in general, the person with AIDS will of course feel it even more than families and friends. It is vital that the person with AIDS should not have to bear the burden of the family's distress. In all this it might be easy to forget that it is the person with AIDS who is the one to suffer the most. It is first and foremost his or her tragedy.

Therefore the family have to learn to accept and cope with the illness themselves in order to be a support to the person with AIDS. He will have quite enough to do sorting his own life without worrying about his family and how they're coping along the way. He'll also be learning how to live with depression, sadness and anger as well as the physical effects of the illness.

Once armed with whatever information is needed, or wanted, and reassured about the low risk of infection, the most important thing for families and friends is to be there when you are needed.

The young man who screwed his courage to the sticking point and told his mother that he was homosexual and also now HIV positive, only to be told by her that she wished she'd "had an abortion", is someone who needs to have superhuman reserves of courage not to be completely devastated. I find it unbelievable that a mother could even think of doing that to a son, but sadly it does happen.

People are often quite young when they are diagnosed as having AIDS, and this causes extra problems. People with AIDS may have to cope with the loss of their job, money problems, housing problems, as well as suffering uncomfortable symptoms. The drugs themselves needed to prolong life and keep certain conditions under control may also make them feel wretched. Families and friends somehow have to find a way of junking past problems or difficulties if there have been some in the past, of forgiving what happened in the past and living in the "now". And admittedly, this is not easy to do when you're suddenly faced with the terror or illness and possibly the death of someone you thought would live into old age.

For the person who is ill it's equally difficult. No one who has been used to living their own life with a degree of independence relishes the thought of being dependent on other people for food, heating and a home.

When a close relative is ill, the tendency is to want to be the one to do the looking after, but the person with AIDS will probably loathe the feeling that their own life is somehow not within their control any more. Family and friends have to learn how to be supportive without taking over, and many people say this is not easy.

It's especially difficult when AIDS affects people living a long way from big cities and their hospitals. In London where many people with AIDS either live or move to, the services are good. *
Every inner London teaching hospital has expert medical care, and special AIDS wards where there is always information about where to get advice or how to join a support group.

There are AIDS units in the hospitals of most of the major cities in Britain. However, if you live in the country miles away from anywhere it is possible to feel very isolated. There may not be an AIDS ward in your local hospital. People with AIDS may well be in the STD (Sexually Transmitted Diseases) or the GU (Genito Urinary) wards where it is difficult to talk openly about the illness.

Many GPs in this country have never met a person with AIDS, and even in London they may only have one or two people with AIDS on their register. So many AIDS patients know more about the disease than their GPs. But since there has been so much written about AIDS over the last five years, most GPs are much more aware of the problem and if they cannot help you much when your relative is diagnosed, then they should at least be able to put you in touch with a local counselling service.

* 70 per cent of AIDS cases are in London. There are hardly any cases in Northern Ireland, in parts of Wales, in Orkney or Shetland, and some areas of rural England.

CARING FOR SOMEONE WITH AIDS

If you are caring for someone with HIV, it is obviously sensible to take precautions in the same way you would if you were caring for someone with hepatitis. It is technically possible for the virus to be transmitted if blood from an infected person gets into the body through broken skin, although again the risk is very low and there are very few such recorded incidences.

If you do accidentally stab yourself with a used needle, clean the wound out without sucking, to get the blood flowing out, and wash it with soap and water and cover with antiseptic and plaster.

If you are caring for someone with AIDS and there is a spillage of urine, vomit, faeces (which may contain traces of blood) or blood itself, clean it up as quickly as possible with a solution of 1 in 10 bleach and hot water. The washing machine will deal with soiled sheets or clothes, using ordinary washing powder. The heat of a hot wash cycle will kill the virus. When clearing up, it is sensible to wear rubber gloves.

Make sure you look after yourself if you're looking after someone with AIDS. Don't take on more than you think you can cope with, give yourself regular breaks and recognise if you're getting stressed so that you can plan ahead. Remember you won't be of much help to your relative if you aren't functioning very well.

There are support services you can call on if you are looking after someone at home. It's important to talk to the person with AIDS about how they may feel if you organise a rota of people to come in to help you out. Many people do not want lots of different "outsiders" streaming in and out, but others will be happy to accept this support if it means staying out of hospital or a hospice.

District nurses are attached to a general practice, so a person with AIDS would have to be registered with a GP to ask for their services. Specialist district or community nurses can come in and give baths, change dressings, and put you in touch with local voluntary services or social services.

Your GP, your local hospital or district nurse can put you in touch with your local Macmillan nursing team. They are trained to care for terminally ill patients, and they are also trained to provide counselling. Your GP or district nurse can also put you in touch with the local hospice, and with DDUs (Drug Dependency Units) should you require them.

Occupational therapists work from hospitals and social services departments, and can help with equipment, such as arranging handles to make getting in and out of the bath easier, providing wheelchairs, or adapting telephones.

You can often arrange a home help, who can do domestic things like laundry and shopping. In many areas there is an HIV AIDS co-ordinator whom you can contact to organise this. The social worker at the hospital will also put you in touch with home helps.

There are many voluntary organisations which provide help and support for those people with AIDS and the people who are looking after them. ACET (AIDS Care Education and Training) have trained nurses who will come and assess the person with AIDS and then provide volunteers to come in on a regular basis and help by preparing a meal, organising an outing, or simply just being around for an hour or two. ACET works on a more or less nationwide basis (see page 215).

Your local Law Centre (if there still is one in your area) or the Citizens Advice Bureau will help if you need a solicitor. The Terrence Higgins Trust will help you make a will, arrange a Power of Attorney, or organise a "Living Will", a legally valid document setting out a person's wishes about terminal care.

BENEFITS AVAILABLE FOR THOSE WITH HIV AND AIDS

Benefits do vary according to personal situations, It is always advisable to enquire at your local DHSS office about what benefits you or your relative are entitled to. If the person with HIV or AIDS is employed or self employed and is able to work, he can claim:

Family Credit
Housing Benefit
Disability Living Allowance

If they are employed but not able to work they will need a sick note from their GP and can claim:

Statutory Sick Pay
Sickness Benefits
Income Support
Housing Benefit
Disability Living Allowance
Social Fund Payments

If they are unemployed, fit for work and are up-to-date with their National Insurance contributions, they can claim:

Unemployment Benefit
Income Support
Housing Benefit
Disability Living Allowance
Social Fund Payments

If they are unemployed but not fit for work and are up-to-date with National Insurance stamps, they will need a sick note from their GP and can claim:

Sickness Benefit
Invalidity Benefit (after 28 weeks)
Income Support
Housing Benefit
Disability Living Allowance
Social Fund Payment

If they have been out of work for some time and have not paid enough National Insurance, they can claim:

Income Support
Housing Benefit
Disability Living Allowance
Social Fund Payments
and possibly severe disablement allowance

A social worker will be able to help your relative to claim these benefits. It is not possible to get the disability living allowance (which incorporates the old attendance allowance and mobility allowance) for the first three months of an illness unless your GP is willing to write a special medical report for the DSS in which he describes the person with AIDS as "terminally ill".

The mobility component is given to people who find it hard to balance, who are unable to walk, or who find walking painful, exhausting, or if it takes a long time. A disabled sticker for the car entitling a person with AIDS to special parking facilities can be obtained through the local council. Special taxi passes are also available from the local council for any taxi journey within a certain radius at a fixed cost of a couple of pounds.

There are special one-off community care grants available from the DSS to provide things without which a person with AIDS might have to go into hospital, or to make it possible for a person to come out of hospital and return home. For example, money for a washing machine or tumble drier, special bedding, kitchen equipment, or money to pay re-connection charges if the power supply has been cut off.

The Motability scheme may help with transport. You will have to contact the Citizens Advice Bureau or the local council if housing is required.

WHAT TO DO IF YOUR RELATIVE DIES

Those with relatives who have died in hospital will find that the hospital will know the procedure for dealing with the body and the formalities. The staff in AIDS wards of hospitals are extremely kind and experienced.

The stories of people in this book whose relatives and friends finished their lives in the Mildmay Mission Hospital, one of the few hospices for people with AIDS, the London Lighthouse or in hospital, show with deep feeling how much was done for them by the staff, both in terms of practical help and emotional and loving support. The local home care team will support families through a death at home, and they are equally skilled in terms of support and advice.

It is possible (though less likely these days) to discover at the last minute that the local undertakers will not deal with the body of a person who has died from an AIDS-related illness, even though if they are members of the National Association of Funeral Directors they should. The distress caused by this can be avoided by using the undertakers recommended by the hospital or the local HIV nurse or home care team.

For families living outside big cities it is sensible to make enquiries locally to make sure there isn't an upsetting hitch at this stage. It is helpful to know that there is a guideline that the body of a person with AIDS has to be put into a zipped body bag, made of heavy plastic. Once the body is in place, and the family and friends have finished their goodbyes, the guidelines state that the bag should not be unzipped again. Elsewhere in the EC this doesn't have to be done. Staff in hospitals and hospices are very sensitive to the distress that this may cause, and will usually make every effort to deal with the body discreetly, perhaps after the relatives have gone home.

People who have been on Income Support or Housing Benefit qualify for financial assistance for the funeral from the DSS. The social worker will be the person to advise families and friends of the deceased. If there is no money at all to pay for a funeral, the local authority will arrange it.

AIDS AND THE FUTURE

At the moment there is still no vaccine against either HIV or AIDS. There is no cure and no wonder drug. In April 1993 scientists declared that trials over some years had proved that the drug AZT was effective for a much shorter time than had previously been thought. Certainly people with HIV and AIDS are living longer than in the early 1980s, but this may well have more to do with the new, more powerful and effective drugs used to treat the separate illnesses which are being developed and refined all the time. As the drugs get more sophisticated the side effects can at the same time be catered for by other drugs, so an AIDS patient can find himself chomping through as many as thirty or forty pills each day.

It took Princess Diana to show the world that we should not be afraid of being with people with AIDS. If we all know exactly what the risks are, and are very clear about what is safe, we ought to be able to get rid of some of the stigma which is attached to the idea of AIDS.

Ignorance breeds fear, and it's a natural reaction to be frightened of the unknown. But once we all know what is involved, then we should all be able to be more open about it with each other, and in the communities in which we live.

AIDS

We are stretched to meet a new dimension
Of love, a more demanding range
Where despair and hope must intertwine.
How grow to meet it? Intention
Here can neither move nor change
The raw truth. Death is on the line.
It comes to separate and estrange
Lover from lover in some reckless design.
Where do we go from here?

Fear. Fear. Fear. Fear.

Our world has never been more stark
Or more in peril.
It is very lonely now in the dark.
Lonely and sterile.

And yet in the simple turn of a head
Mercy lives. I heard it when someone said
"I must go now to a dying friend.
Every night at nine I tuck him into bed,
And give a shot of morphine,"
And added, "I go where I have never been."
I saw he meant into a new discipline
He had not imagined before, and a new grace.

Every day now we meet it face to face.
Every day now devotion is the test.
Through the long hours, the hard, caring nights
We are forging a new union. We are blest.

As closed hands open to each other
Closed lives open to strange tenderness
We are learning the hard way to mother.
Who says it is easy? But we have the power.
I watch the faces deepen all around me.
It is the time of change, the saving hour.
The word is not fear, the word we live,
But an old world suddenly made new,
As we learn it again, as we bring it alive:

Love. Love. Love. Love.

May Sarton

2
The Stories

Dany and Michael Sheils lived together in London for sixteen years. Michael worked as a reporter with BBC Radio, finally working on the Radio 4 programme The World Tonight. *Dany works as an accountant in the West End of London. They met when Dany came over from France on a one-year training course in London, and formed a relationship which they both were certain would be lifelong.*

DANY

I met Michael in November 1973 and he died in February 1989, in our sixteenth year. I arrived in London in September 1973, so I'd been here about six weeks – not long – and I had plans to be here just for one year to learn English and then to go back to France, and then I met him and that was it. I was born in Brittany and I still have both my parents and a brother who live there. I also have a sister who lives in Paris who is married with three children. Her little boy was born on Michael's death anniversary, the 24th February 1991 and that was lovely because then I felt the cycle was closed, death, departure, new arrival.

I was very lucky because we always had a large circle of friends, most of whom worked at the BBC and we'd been accepted as a couple for many many years.

We decided to tell just a few people that Michael was HIV. Those people were our closest friends and that really helped me because we did not tell his mother, for instance, and we didn't tell my family either. Just those few friends, about eight in all. And Michael didn't say anything at work because it was in 1987 and he was still working there, and we didn't know how the BBC would react – all those question marks! So we kept it quiet for a while, but it was a very heavy weight to carry. Life went on, but as far as we were concerned – the two of us – a drama was being played and time was running short. Yet we had to survive, and to be quite strong and positive and make the most of it.

The first sign that something was wrong was after Michael returned from a trip to the Seychelles. He'd been away a couple of weeks, and he came back with shingles. I remember he was really ill – he had to crawl from his bedroom to the bathroom.

I was working at the Cumberland Hotel at the time and because we lived close by I used to come back at lunch-time to check on him. I couldn't believe he was really that ill – so I was quite hard on him, you know, telling him to come on and get up. It took a long long time for me to realise that he was really very ill, and that changed everything. From that time on he began to age and to lose weight, although he recovered a little bit from the shingles. But there was always something else.

He had a very bad eye for a long time, not just for a few months but for almost a year. The infection wouldn't go away, and then he wouldn't eat very much and he was always tired. I can't remember everything he got, but there was always something. I remember we went to Provence in September 1986, before the shingles in fact, and he had this bad eye and couldn't see properly. He had to lie down before we did anything – it got quite boring, you know, considering we were on holiday!

So after a few months of being quite ill I began to wonder what was wrong with him. And I thought of HIV. We didn't discuss it, but it was on my mind and I think it must have been on his as well. And after a while we agreed maybe he should take a test. Michael was always very strong, very brave, and very independent. He went for the test and got the result by himself, and then he told me. And when he told me I must say I wasn't surprised, but it was a terrible blow because from the minute he told me I knew our life would never be the same again, never again. And also, I had to think about myself as well, you know?

We had a lovely doctor at the Middlesex Hospital, and he said "One thing at a time, you can have your test later. Let's cope with Michael being ill first of all." So we waited, but of course it was on my mind all the time whether I was OK. Was I going to be ill one day too?

So six months later I asked to have the test. And I was so frightened, really frightened, but I was negative. I've had two more tests since and I've just had a third last week. The second one

50

was three years later so I should be fine. I knew I probably would be because of our style of life, but who knows really and I don't know how I would cope if I were to become positive. Because having gone through it all with Michael I know what it represents. And he was lucky to have me. I've got nobody.

Michael was diagnosed in February 1987 and after that there always seemed to be something wrong. He never seemed to have the chance to get well again, even for a short period. During the next two years there was never a week where we could dream for a bit and think it was all some awful nightmare.

You'd never know that some people are HIV – they're still working, and they're healthy, leading a normal life. We never had that. Maybe it was because he was a bit older – he was forty-four when he got ill.

To begin with there was a lot of anger, a lot of anger from me – I was hurt, obviously, and I was very angry with him. Because you know in those days, after all, he was one of the experts on AIDS in BBC radio.

Any time there was news about HIV and AIDS, it would be Michael who was asked to report. He followed the Health Minister, Norman Fowler, to Los Angeles to view the hospitals and see what they were doing there. That was in the early 1980s and Michael was there! So I was very angry that he knew more than most other people, and yet he got it. It wasn't that he'd been unfaithful, I could cope with that, it was that he bloody got it. So not only was he going to die and destroy his life, but he was destroying our life too.

And for a long time I wanted to leave, I wanted to escape. I wasn't going to waste my time, waste my life waiting for him to die – I wanted to leave. And I told him so. Looking back, that makes me sad – I was being very cruel, very selfish. And when it came to it, I couldn't do it.

Later on, the fact that Michael had been unfaithful to me and caught the virus took second or even third place because all we could do and think about was what life was like for him now, never mind where he got it, with whom, when or how. I couldn't have cared less.

It had happened anyway, and it was too late to reflect on that.

The questions were what did we do now, how did we survive, what could we do next?

I coped with my anger by coming to my senses, I suppose, and realising what we had got. We'd had a long, successful and fruitful partnership, and I very quickly understood that my part to play in all this was to help Michael, and love him, and support him as much as I could. I could never, never, have left him, never.

For a while after he was diagnosed he was angry too, maybe not so much for having got the virus, but more for having destroyed all he'd got, which was us as a couple and the happiness we had shared for so long. Because there was no question in our minds about us, we were well together, settled, and were going to spend the rest of our lives together, it was good. But I think he must have felt very, very guilty. Later on in the illness I know he talked to the priest at the Mildmay, to try and come to terms with his guilt. I don't know what was said, but I know it took him a long time to deal with what was said.

He carried on working for quite a little while, but it became more and more difficult. At lunch-time, because we live so close, he would pretend to come back for lunch here but in fact he would come home to go to bed. And he would take longer and longer lunchbreaks. And as the illness became more and more visible, they were not fools, they understood, but they were quiet. They respected the fact that he was being discreet.

His last broadcast was on Worlds AIDS Day 1987, which was about him having the illness. It was a brilliant piece of broadcasting. We had an amazing response from people who knew his name, who knew his work, and especially loved his beautiful voice; they wrote to him and to us, showing their love and affection, and telling us how sorry they were. And that Christmas we wrote back to everyone. There were plans to do another piece following his progress, but his first broadcast was so moving, almost like a farewell, you could never follow something like that. We agreed that would be that, and it turned out to be his last piece of journalism and he stopped work after that. So he must have told the BBC not long after he'd been diagnosed.

He was very thin and gaunt, and little by little he became like an old man, always tired and wanting to sleep all the time. He was on AZT for a little while, but I think he was too far gone for that to have much effect. He had a lot of diarrhoea and then the difficult bit was having to realise that he was not in control of his bodily functions any more, and very quickly he was stuck.

He couldn't plan to do anything or go anywhere because he wasn't sure he'd be able to cope with his body. That was a terrible part of the illness.

Although Michael was very strong and positive he was also very realistic at times and he knew that his days were numbered. He would often say "I'm finished, I'm finished". And that's very difficult to cope with, when someone is dying. What do you say? It still breaks my heart to look back and remember him saying those words.

He was in and out of the Middlesex – I can't remember exactly why or what happened, I think I've elected to blot all that out from my mind. The time did come when the Community Care team from the Middlesex intervened, but not until quite late in his life, about January 1989. By then he was having to inject himself, and he had a tube coming out of his heart. When I look back, it was awful to see that tube coming out of his body. He was injecting himself – and I couldn't do it, and he wanted to do it himself anyway. But it got so that he couldn't do it, he was trembling too much, and there was the danger of getting air bubbles and I got very frightened. So the Community Care team came round to do it for him.

But they obviously realised he was getting towards the end, so they took him first into the Middlesex and then they transferred him to the Mildmay. But they didn't tell me, openly, what they were doing – they just said the Mildmay would be a good idea. That they were very well equipped and had all the right drugs, that he could go there for a bit and then maybe come home, and I swallowed everything, I believed them.

I wonder now whether they really knew or not it was coming to the end. But I think that Michael knew that somehow the time had come to go either to the Lighthouse or to the Mildmay, and I think he must have known. And I think it was a kind of relief, in a way; a relief that he was going to be taken care of medically and that it would not involve me, because he always wanted to keep

53

his independence and his dignity. He was very strong and very positive. He looked after himself really, I didn't do very much. But he knew that he couldn't do it any more.

So John, a friend, drove him to the Mildmay, and from the moment he got there, he felt better, he felt at peace. He stayed there for four weeks before he died.

From the time he was diagnosed, Michael, being what he was and who he was, was also very concerned about me and my future.

We discussed what I should do and we thought that I would go back to France after he died. So he helped me to prepare to go back to France. We had a large cottage in Norfolk, and a tiny house in Provence, and the idea was to sell the cottage in Norfolk and buy something bigger in France where I could start again. So we did that together, although basically I did the practical things.

And I'm glad we had the time to sell the cottage and do that together. We found this lovely, lovely house in Provence which I still have, and we had the time to move, to go there a few times together, and he was able to put his mark on the house. That to him was important, because he knew that at least I'd got a lovely place to go back to. It was something outside the illness, and it kept us very busy. It was good.

We told his mother on his birthday in October 1988. She was living in Cheshire and she came down to London. We felt by then that time was running short and that she should know. His father was dead, his brother lived in Tasmania and his sister lived in the Cayman Islands. His sister knew, though, we'd told her the first summer after he was diagnosed. She used to come back with her family every summer and they'd stay in the cottage in Norfolk, and the cottage would become the family home for a few weeks. Michael's mother would join us too.

Michael's mother is an extraordinary lady really, and somehow she coped. She knew all about us – it was all in the open – and we had a very good relationship. We'd take her to Provence and she would come to the cottage, she knew all our friends, and she was really part of our lives. We called her Granny. But still we were very frightened to tell her, because we knew it would be very painful for her. She was due to spend that winter with her daughter in the Cayman Islands, but she didn't want to leave Michael – we had to push her a little bit into going.

When he moved into the Mildmay I would visit Michael every day but I quickly became very frightened, he looked so awful. He was also very thin, and I could see death in his eyes. He was beginning to become blind and he was very frightened of that. He gradually saw less and less, and he was very very weak and looked a typical AIDS patient. Drugs were poured into him and he was eating nothing.

Michael went into the Mildmay on the Friday and on the Sunday John, who'd driven him in, rang me and said, "Look Dany, I really don't think it looks good." I agreed with him and so I asked the doctor (of the Community Care team) whether I should call the family, but he said there was plenty of time and I should wait. Looking back, I was by myself and it was a difficult decision to make – all the weight was on my shoulders. Because, I said to myself, if I didn't call them it might be too late, and if I did call them and it's a false alarm I'm going to worry them for nothing. After all they were coming from the Cayman Islands and Tasmania!

In the end I said I didn't care, time was really running short and I asked Michael, "Do you want to see them?" And he said, "I leave it to you." So I did ring them, and I was so pleased that I did. Of course it took them days to arrive here, by the time they'd booked the flight and everything. So in the end they had three weeks with him. The first week he was still good, he pushed himself a little bit and saw them for a few hours each day. They'd go during the day, and I'd go by myself in the evening so he had time with his family on his own. They told me that he'd sit on his bed and he'd hold a sort of meeting with his family! He was trying to persuade his mother to move back to Ireland where she came from – he said, Mother, you must do it – he was very strong.

He was often in pain – I think he put on a little bit of show at first for the family, but by the time I got there after work, he was exhausted and could hardly talk. We both had a religious faith. I knew I had to prepare for the death and the funeral, and about a month before Michael died I went to St James's Church in Spanish Place. We'd been going to Mass there quite regularly, so they must have seen us. After Mass one day, I asked to see the main priest, Mgr Miles, and I made an appointment and went two days later to see him in his office.

I was a bit frightened, because I needed his help. I knew I wanted a proper funeral Mass, and it would have been nice to have used that beautiful church where we'd both been. So I explained who I was, who we were, and what had happened. But I could feel and see the hostility from the beginning, and I knew it was a lost cause. First of all he let me talk, but he was reluctant to do anything about it. I think he was afraid to be seen by the neighbourhood and the people who went to Mass to be doing anything about AIDS.

I got quite angry with him and asked him whether that was really the church he was representing. I gave him a second chance, and I really pushed him, but he wouldn't budge. He left me with a very heavy burden to carry. He didn't even make any suggestions about where I could go next.

In the end it was a nun who worked at the Middlesex who helped me. She'd known Michael there and came to visit him at the Mildmay. She and the priest of the church she was attached to decided between them that they would help me.

In the end, Michael faded away, gently and slowly. Somehow I think having seen his family, and shown them he wasn't too bad, he thought, well now's the time, I've seen them, I can let go. It was a beautiful death actually. I even had the time to call our very close friends, and they all came in and he was able to have proper goodbyes with everybody.

That was on the Sunday, and from that day I said no more friends, the remaining time is for us, the family. So from then till the Friday when he died, there were just the four of us, his mother, sister, brother and myself.

Michael was afraid to die by himself – he wanted me especially to be with him, so for the last week we were there on call twenty-four hours a day. So two of us would sleep at the Mildmay and they provided sleeping arrangements. They were wonderful. I feel very grateful that being a Frenchman, in England, in those early days of AIDS, I was so well looked after, that I was privileged to have people who understood, who cared, and who loved us and who

56

showed it as well. And there was no problem for me to be part of a gay couple, it seemed absolutely normal, there was no added pressure.

I was on duty on the last night; everyone is in private rooms at the Mildmay, and they put a bed ready for me by the side of his bed for me to sleep on. And we were exhausted, all of us. I went to talk to him, and he didn't respond very much, but I knew maybe he could hear me. And I almost said, Michael, look, let it go, please, let it go, I can't cope with any more, please go. And he died quite soon after.

Now I look back on Michael's death, and it was a beautiful death, and I was lucky to be there in the few minutes it happened. And while it was happening, and after it happened, there was, surprisingly, a lot of joy – a great deal of joy because I saw, I witnessed, the passage from life to death. I saw it and I felt it. It was a relief in a way, we'd had time to prepare, and it came peacefully, slowly.

In the last few days, Michael was in a coma. In fact it's amazing because he went into the coma the day after he'd said goodbye to his closest friends. I really feel he was ready, he wasn't fighting any more.

There does come a time when there is no more energy left to fight. Michael was always a very strong guy, very hopeful, very positive, and that helped him a lot, because if you're like that you can fight back a bit. I wouldn't be like that, I think I'd be dead before I began!

Michael died on Friday late afternoon, and there were four people present; his sister Moira, Father Tim, the Catholic priest from the Mildmay who Michael liked very much, Sister Anna, and myself. Mrs Sheils was resting; she had had a difficult day. Patrick, Michael's brother, had decided to return to Tasmania that day after three weeks in London. He called us from the airport just before catching the plane, at the precise time Michael died. Father Tim took the call and said to Patrick, "Both of you will travel tonight." I thought that was a beautiful thing to say to the brother, who was very upset not to be there, having "waited" all that time. Imagine flying all the way to Tasmania, alone, having just lost your brother.

I remember that Princess Diana came to visit the Mildmay the day of Michael's death; we saw her, and her entourage passed by Michael's bedroom.

We couldn't do anything over the weekend, but they gave us an outline of what we should do on the Monday. It was all very straightforward – Veronica Moss, the doctor, delivered the death certificate, and suggested a firm of undertakers. So we went back on the Monday to collect the death certificate, and they told us where to go to register the death. And then the Catholic priest at the Mildmay joined us at the flat, and I felt quite well prepared.

I think it is very important for anybody, whether in a relationship or not, to prepare for death as fully as possible. For instance, Michael said to me, "I leave everything to you Dany; only two things. I don't want any flowers, and I want my ashes to be put in the garden in Provence." Those were the only two things. He trusted me completely, so I did everything. I'm a good organiser. And I wanted a funeral which was for both of us in a way. We never had a proper wedding, so I wanted the funeral to be special, to be something very personal. I rang everyone to tell them – I wanted everyone to be there. And everybody was there. I wanted my family to be there, and they all came over, all nine of them.

My sister and my brother knew exactly what our relationship had been, so did my parents; we never discussed it because from the time I met Michael I never went back to my parents without him, and we shared the same bedroom. He was part of the family there, and they loved him. So nothing was said, but it was accepted. It was lovely to have the two families and all the friends together.

The church was full, it was a poignant service, and I came in leading the two families, with Michael's mother on my arm, and I led them on the way out as well. Our friends Jilly and Sally read the lessons, Wendy read the poem by Canon Scott Holland, and Sheelagh sang "Thou art my Joy" by J S Bach. Other close friends welcomed everybody at the entrance of the church, and made sure that everyone signed the "Guest Book". The priest in the sermon mentioned the obituary in *The Independent*, written by the Editor of *The World Tonight*, and he also talked about us as a couple, and mentioned me by name – I feel very privileged about that. I wanted to have contact with everyone, so I shook hands with everyone, that was important to me.

After the Requiem Mass in Soho there was a private cremation, with only the two families and the very close friends. Then a group of us went out to the Cumberland Hotel and we had a splendid meal to celebrate Michael's life.

I know Michael would have liked that. And one friend suddenly got up and sang a verse of the Edith Piaf song, "Je ne regrette rien", and I asked my father to sing one of his songs in response, which he did. He'd always done that at parties in France, so Michael knew his songs well.

Everything was in order. Michael prepared very well, he made a list, so the will, the insurance, everything was done. And he talked to his family about the will. It was very important to him that there would be no problems later on. He wanted to give me his estate, his full estate, and he wanted them to know, and they understood and agreed. One does hear awful stories about families fighting after the death.

The other thing he wanted to arrange was for his mother and I to carry on looking after each other, and he made us promise we would look after each other, and we have. In fact, I've coped with it all because my best counsellor was his mother. She was here three weeks before his death, and afterwards, when his brother and sister went back home, she elected to stay with me for about two months, and she stayed here in the flat with me. I think I love her more now than I love my own mother. I can talk to her about anything, anything, and I'm glad she stayed with me then. We cried together and we talked about it, and she looked after me.

I remember someone suggesting I should perhaps go and see a professional bereavement counsellor. He was a professional man and I'm sure he had lots of experience, yet he was so cold, so distant, so indifferent. I was meant to be there for an hour, but after five minutes, I thought, "What am I here for? Who is that man? I don't need him, I'm going back to Granny." And I didn't need anybody else.

Granny now lives in Armagh. When she went back to Ireland she was very concerned about what people would say to her, and especially what they would think. She found it difficult to tell them what Michael died of and she was very worried about it. In fact a lot of people had heard Michael's broadcast, and people in the end were all right about it, but she still worried about it a lot. After all, she's an older lady, in her eighties now, and she was going back to the same place where she had been a doctor's wife after ten or twenty years, so she did feel a bit pressurised.

At work I never came out. I felt that my way of doing things was just to get on with life and be normal, I didn't feel there was any need to tell everyone about my private life. But things became very difficult – I remember how it felt to be at work with this burden of Michael getting iller, and feeling like screaming, and crying. I had to pretend, and that was very difficult.

I did eventually tell my boss, just before Michael went into the Mildmay. He understood, I think maybe he had guessed. And he said I could take as much time off as I wanted. So I went to my doctor and got the necessary sick note, because officially I was supposed to be off sick. And in the end I was away from work for about a month, and they were very good about it. The accounts office where I worked was a large one, and the deputy chief accountant and another colleague came to the funeral, and when I came back they were very gentle, very gentle with me. So although not very much was said openly, they understood and treated me very well.

The BBC themselves were good to me as well – they rang me up before the death, and I went to see someone in Personnel. They knew about the long relationship I'd had with Michael, and they really treated me like a wife or husband, like a real partner. They asked if financially I was OK, if I needed anything I was to let them know, and they wanted to do something for me. They wanted to arrange some sort of pension for me, although in the end that wasn't possible.

So they gave me a large sum of money which covered the expense of the funeral. Michael had always been a freelance and therefore not entitled to a staff pension. I thought it was extraordinary – I'd never have asked them for money and I found it amazing that they should want to look after me in that way.

I also realise we were lucky to live in the middle of London. At one stage we played with the idea of selling the flat and going to live in Norfolk but we decided it was out of the question – our flat was close to the Middlesex, one of the best hospitals for AIDS, with all the drugs and the care we needed.

And even now, after the result of my third HIV test last week, I wondered what would I do if I was positive? Because I'm planning to return to France in a few years' time, or at least when I get to retirement time. But if I was HIV positive, I'm not so sure I would do that, I think I'd remain in London.

I feel it's vital for someone who is losing a partner to encourage their friends and neighbours to talk to them about it. I'm very good at that – even now, four years later, I still talk about it a lot. I'm always talking about Michael and it's always me that starts the subject. People feel more at ease if I've been the one to start the conversation. It was very important to me too that people wrote such lovely letters to me, that was really helpful.

By far the most significant thing in all this has been the way we've been treated with love and dignity, not accusingly as gays, or as drug addicts or whatever. Michael was treated as a human being who was going to die, and we were helped to come to terms with this, to accept it and to find peace. I think that's what the Mildmay, the family, the friends, did for Michael. We all joined in and in that sense he was very lucky, as a gay person in the eighties, to die with all that love. In a way you could say that my story is an ideal one in the sense that as a gay couple we were accepted, there was no extra pressure put on us because of our gayness or the HIV. I feel sad for the single gay guy who has got HIV and who has not only to cope with the illness, which is a real drama, but with the notion that he can't tell his family, or he can't tell his neighbours, I had none of that. And that's why I feel a great debt to society, and that's why I'm still in touch with the Mildmay. I've applied to be part of the voluntary team – I want to do something. I want to help somebody to die peacefully the way Michael died, because it was a privilege to be at the Mildmay.

COLIN *was one of seven children. He lived by himself in a council flat in Whitechapel and did a variety of office jobs. His family had guessed that he was gay, but Colin himself refused to admit this to his family. His mother was a widow. He died in the Mildmay Hospice, supported by all his family including his elder brother Paul and sister-in-law Sarah.*

PAUL

Colin always pretended he had girl friends, even to the extent of having our parents round to supper and pretending that his girlfriend couldn't be there because of a crisis at home. I think he thought they would react very badly if he told them he was gay. We've talked about it since he died and my mother, although she recognised that one or two of his friends were gay, says it honestly never occurred to her that Colin might be gay.

Mum works in a hospital so she's interested in disease, and could go into detail about lots of illnesses. But she seemed to have blocked AIDS out of her mind.

Colin went on holiday to France with one of our sisters and her husband and they noticed that he had trouble walking – his legs didn't seem to be working properly, and he was losing a lot of weight.

I run my own business and he came to do some assembly work for me that summer, because he hadn't got a regular job at the time, and he seemed very slow and unco-ordinated. He had a real struggle to do quite easy things. I suggested a few times that he should go and see a doctor, but he'd just fly off the handle. His defence was always aggression, he'd always snap at you rather than explain things, that was his way of dealing with everything.

I picked Colin up one weekend from Mum's and he looked dreadful. He said he'd fallen down the stairs – Sarah thought he'd been beaten up because several times in the past he'd come back with black eyes and bruises. Anyway, he'd hurt his chest so I took him to casualty, and all that happened was that we waited around for six hours only to be told he should go and see his own doctor.

It was very difficult to help him – when we were at Mum's at weekends he'd tell us that he had a job, even telling us stories

62

about things that happened at work. Then he'd go back to the flat on Monday and not eat because he didn't have any money.

At the New Year we were all together at Mum's, and he was really difficult. Nothing was right, he criticised everything. Later he tried to stand up to go to the loo and his legs gave way. By this time we all knew we'd got to do something about it. It was very difficult because he was always saying he'd been up to the hospital, that they'd said it was this or that, or that they'd done tests.

Sarah was certain it was AIDS, although we hadn't known anyone with it. So we phoned the National Aids Helpline, just to get some idea of what we could do. When we described his condition they did say it sounded as if it could be AIDS, and that we should really get him to see somebody. I went to the flat to see him on his own, and brought up the subject of AIDS. I found it almost impossible to do. He'd built up this protective wall around him, so it was always hard to talk to him.

Before Christmas I'd made a point of going down to the flat once or twice a week at lunch-time, to take him out for a drink and play a game of snooker, which was extremely difficult for me, what with trying to find the time inbetween running my own company. But I did it to try and get some sort of bridge established. But when I confronted him about his illness, he just reacted with total anger. He stormed out and said "You'd better go," and I said, "Come on Colin, we need to sit down. This isn't going to go away, and we need to see if there's something we can do about it," and he put his coat on and went to the front door. Then he suddenly turned round and came back, and said "Well, all right, then."

He'd obviously been bottling it up for months, and he realised things weren't getting better. Afterwards he said he had got friends who'd died from AIDS, so it had obviously crossed his mind, and he knew he was at risk and he was frightened. So he agreed to go for a test. He'd been to the STD clinic at the Whitechapel Hospital on some previous occasion, and he said he'd go back there. Later he told me he had an appointment, and he showed us the letter. We wrote down the doctor's name and telephone number – I know it sounds awful to have resorted to that but he'd told us so many fibs.

I had an HIV test later because of the cuts and grazes Colin and I

63

both got while we worked together on the assembly line. I'm a blood donor and I didn't want to risk anything. I went to the local HIV clinic, and I had my counselling first. I had to explain why I wanted it, and I felt they were definitely there to talk me out of it – they seemed to have lots of reasons why I shouldn't have the test. I deliberately didn't go to my GP, in case the fact I'd asked for a test might go against me when it came to medicals for life insurance or something. All that side of it makes seeking an HIV test seem very furtive and seedy. I had two tests some months apart and they were clear.

By this time Colin was piling up huge amounts of debt on different bank accounts and it was getting to be a desperate situation. He was behind with the rent too. I paid him to work weekends to help him out, and I felt that made us a bit closer. We said that if he told us the extent of his problems we'd see if we could sort out something. One day though we went round to his flat and discovered the phone was about to be cut off, and we were concerned about that because he was living on the tenth floor of a tower block and anything could have happened – he could have collapsed. His phone bill turned out to be for hundreds of pounds, and he was meant to be paying it off every month. Sarah tried for hours to get the phone company to allow him to go on paying it off, but they just said no way, and that if he got cut off the reconnection charge would have to be paid in full and they would insist on a deposit. So the phone was cut off.

Then we rang up the clinic to check on whether he'd been for the test, and they said they weren't allowed to disclose information because of confidentiality. We explained that we'd been trying to get him down there, and so they told us he had been there, they remembered him, but he'd refused to have the test. The clinic said that they didn't need him to take the test to know that he had got AIDS, he was so far gone. But of course they couldn't start any treatment until he had tested positive.

Later Colin told us he'd had the test, and he would get the results the following week. We couldn't say anything, so we left it. Then he told us he'd got the result and he was all right. So then I finally confronted him – it was blackmail really – I said to him, "Is that the honest truth then Colin? Because look, I'm a blood donor, I'm going to give blood next Monday, so if what you're telling me is right there are no problems, but if there's any doubt at all, I don't want to go and give blood." So then he admitted to me that he hadn't had the test.

He went the following week and came up to tell us that the test was positive. I would have been quite happy to discuss his homosexuality with him then, but he couldn't talk about it. Even when he told us he was HIV positive, he said "I'm not gay, I'm bisexual." He still didn't want to be known as gay.

Although he was devastated to find out that he had AIDS, he was also very positive about starting the treatment. We discussed with him whether he should tell the rest of the family; but he was against anyone else knowing, especially Mum. We weren't happy about that, but we did feel we had to respect his wishes. We were hoping that over the coming months we would be able to persuade him to tell the rest of the family.

The hospital put him on a high dose of AZT, at once, on the Thursday, and his character totally changed overnight. At the weekend he was meant to be coming over to Mum's. He phoned me on Saturday morning to say he'd got to Wood Green and he didn't have any money. I went to collect him and he was completely spaced out. He'd got a holdall with him into which he'd packed some very strange things. He'd been violently sick. We didn't know this, but with AZT it's very important to take it every four hours, even to setting the alarm clock for the early hours of the morning, otherwise there are dreadful side effects. We didn't know whether he'd overdosed on the stuff. He had the carton of AZT pills, and it seemed to be half empty.

I dropped him off at Mum's. Mum still didn't know he'd had the test, but we said if he was going to stay with her she had to know, in case he was sick or something else happened. But he wouldn't let us tell her. We went over again on the Sunday. He'd often go to Mum's at the weekend to cut the grass or the hedge and he had this thing in his head that he wanted to do that this weekend. When we arrived Mum was tearing her hair out.

Colin hadn't been able to get the electric lawnmower going, so for some reason he'd cut the lead off it, and then he'd tried to do the hedge and couldn't get the hedge-cutter going. So he'd taken the lead off that and instead of wiring them back to the plugs, he'd wired the two together. He'd put the uncovered plug without the cover on it in the main socket, how he didn't get electrocuted I don't know. I looked at him and said, "Colin, what are you doing?" I took him through it and he just couldn't see what he'd done wrong, and all round the house he'd taken the plugs off all the appliances, there were bits everywhere. Then he said he'd got a headache, and we put him to bed. We still didn't know whether to say anything to Mum, so we went home to think about what to do.

In the evening we got a phone call from Mum to say Colin had just collapsed. It's ten minutes down the road, so we dashed round. He was still on the floor, although he was conscious, and I lifted him and put him on the chair and said to him that we needed to get a doctor round. He was totally against that, he wouldn't hear of it, and he still wouldn't let us tell Mum about the illness.

In the end, she was in the kitchen and I just went in and told her, and came back to Colin and said, "It's done now". If the doctor came it was going to come out then so she had to know.

I had said to her before that something was obviously seriously wrong with Colin and what did she think it was? And she would come out with different things, like motor neurone disease. We'd say, "Look it could be HIV," and she just sort of blocked it off. So there we were, trying to get Colin to have a doctor in one room, and Mum trying to come round from what we'd just told her in the other room. She was just in total shock really, she just cried and cried.

We did call the doctor and he was a locum because it was night-time. He was a very nice Australian and he was great. But the situation was that if Colin said he didn't want to go into hospital, there was nothing the doctor could do. He said if Colin changed his mind we should call him again and he would arrange for an ambulance to take him back from Enfield to the Whitechapel. We tried to persuade Colin, but he was absolutely adamant – as far as he was concerned you went into hospital to die and he was not going in. Talking to him afterwards, it was a lot to do with friends – he'd visited them in hospital and they'd never come out.

That night we made a bed up for him in the lounge, because we couldn't change his mind about going to hospital and we couldn't get him upstairs to bed.

It was frightening because it had happened so quickly – he'd only gone to the hospital four days before. And then he'd seemed so much better, and much more positive, and we had felt better because at last he was getting some treatment. The doctors had told him at the clinic that although AZT wouldn't cure him, it might be a good five years before anything happened to him, and then who knows what cures there might be? So to go from that to being sick and totally confused and collapsing a few days later was very frightening. We'd asked the doctor about whether the AZT had caused these symptoms and he didn't really know – he was very sympathetic about the AIDS thing, but he felt Colin needed expert advice.

The next day Mum had to go to work, so I arranged to go over and look after him. The locum doctor the previous day had made arrangements for Mum's doctor to visit in the afternoon. When I arrived Colin had been doubly incontinent and sick; he was in a dreadful state, confused and in a terrible mess. I did what I could for him and then the doctor came. But the doctor just didn't want to know. I'd explained the situation to him and he didn't want to go near him. He just said, "Well Colin you should go into hospital," and Colin said he didn't want to go, and the doctor just turned round to me and said, "Well, there's nothing I can do," and left me. I know now what I would have liked to have said to him and afterwards I wanted to write a letter to him. But at the time there was so much to be done it was difficult to cope. I felt that even if the doctor couldn't have done anything, he could at least have offered to arrange for some support, for someone else to come like a district nurse or someone. But he went, and I didn't know what to do.

I couldn't leave Colin in the state he was in, so I carried him upstairs and gave him a bath. While he was in the bath the phone rang and I went downstairs to answer it. When I got back upstairs, Colin was motionless and completely submerged in the water. I thought he'd drowned. I grabbed hold of his head and pulled him up out of the water. At which point he shouted at me, "What the hell are you doing?". He told me later that he always washed his hair by putting his head under the water to rinse it, but it was certainly a shock we could both have done without. Once we'd finished the bath, he was incontinent again. So I cleaned him up, put new sheets on the bed and tried to make him comfortable. It was all new to me so I just did what seemed right. But I was extremely annoyed by that doctor just leaving me on my own with Colin. Anyway then we knew we just had to get him into hospital.

Sarah came over from work and eventually we talked him into it and he agreed to go. Then we had to ring up the locum doctor again to organise the ambulance. This time we weren't so lucky. It was a different locum and he just didn't want to know. He got extremely stroppy with us and he certainly didn't want to organise an ambulance to take Colin over to the Whitechapel.

So instead we got cross with him – we'd had a really stressful two days, and having spent so much time getting Colin to agree to go into hospital it was pointless for him to end up in the local hospital with no AIDS ward and people not knowing what the situation was. So in the end we just got angry, and the locum had to ring the Whitechapel and get the Accident and Emergency to agree to admit him.

SARAH

At the same time Colin was saying he'd agreed to go to hospital he was adamant he'd go on his own. He wanted particular clothes to take with him, and we knew that what he was planning to do was to get to the hospital and then go round to his flat, which was round the corner. But by this time we were one jump ahead of him. The ambulance guys arrived, and they were very nice – they had to put him in a wheelchair because he couldn't walk. I said to Colin that I'd go with him to see him into the hospital, and we didn't tell him that Paul would follow behind in the car to bring me back.

We got to the hospital at about midnight, and they knew about him and prioritised him so the doctor would see him next. But by four o'clock in the morning we were still sitting in Casualty.

Colin was in a cubicle under the assumption that I'd gone home, and we were outside waiting to see the doctor. When the doctor had seen him she came to see us and said that he was planning to do exactly what we had thought, to leave and go home to his flat. So she'd said to him, "OK, if that's what you want, you can leave." He'd stood up and just collapsed on the floor, so she'd said, "I don't really think you're going anywhere are you?" She told us that she'd got to get him into a ward but she didn't know where, so we should ring in the morning. So about five o'clock in the morning we went home.

About eight o'clock the next morning Mum rang up in a panic. She'd had a phone call from Colin who'd said he was going to get a taxi and to make sure she was at home because he didn't have any money. We rang the hospital and got through to the ward he was in – I think they'd had quite a difficult night with him! Colin was insisting on going home and if he was insisting there wasn't much they could do about it, they'd have to let him go. I said, "You can't let him out, he can't even walk."

The next phone call we got was from Nigel Harvey, the HIV social worker at the Hospital. He'd been called in to try and sort Colin out. At one point Colin had managed to get himself to an internal phone, dialled 999 and had apparently ordered an ambulance to take him out of hospital, which started all the machinery working, of course. Paul had meetings all that day so I went in that afternoon to see Nigel Harvey who wanted to try and get some more background information about Colin. By this time I think Colin was tying the entire hospital up in knots.

His mental state was quite bad at this stage, but he was still insisting on going home, but the hospital wanted to do a lumbar puncture and a brain scan. Eventually Colin agreed to stay in for another day and have the tests. I think the hospital thought that after that he'd be so weak he would forget about going home. Mum came in and we all went to see him. It wasn't nice, because he was in the isolation ward – there were no other beds, it wasn't anyone's fault. But you had to get into all these gowns, and for Colin it seemed as if everyone was suddenly having to be protected against him.

He'd had the lumbar puncture, which would knock most people out, but he'd got this incredible strength from somewhere and he was up and about, making sure we knew he was going home tomorrow and where all his clothes were. He was totally confused, but he could remember every little thing he wanted to if it was to do with going home.

The lumbar puncture didn't produce anything conclusive, but they said that his brain had shrunk right down and was really very small. Basically the disease had affected his whole nervous system and had got to the brain as well. When we spoke to the doctors they thought he would probably only live a couple of weeks and that he might as well continue with the AZT. There was no point in any other treatment.

The next day we got another phone call from the social worker to say Colin was still insisting on going home and there was nothing they could do about it and had we got his keys! Which of course we had – we'd very carefully not left them with his things in the hospital. We were really concerned about him going home on his own to a tenth-floor tower block. The social worker said he was arranging for the Home Care team from the Mildmay to go in with him, and they'd agreed with the Social Services from Tower Hamlets to provide twenty-four-hour care, which was wonderful.

So off we went to the Whitechapel with the keys. They'd arranged for the psychiatrist to see Colin before he left hospital, to make sure Colin knew exactly what the situation was, that he was going home on the understanding that someone would be with him. So the psychiatrist (who looked more nutty than Colin) said yes, Colin was fine to go home.

So Colin tootled off with the hospital chaplain and the girl from the Mildmay pushing him down the road in his wheelchair to his flat.

PAUL

Then we had a phone call a little later to say that Colin had thrown everyone out of the flat. He'd already told us not to come over that evening because he was going out for a drink! I was really concerned – what if he turned the gas on and blew up the flat, or collapsed? So I went rushing over there. I rang on his bell but there was no answer. I rang a few times and then a little later he came to the door. How he managed to get himself there I don't know. I asked him to open the door, and he said he couldn't, it was locked.

I didn't know whether he was just lying to get rid of me, or what. He told me the people had gone out to get some keys cut and he was locked in. I was going spare by this time, and then the Home Care people came back with the keys and I realised they had locked him in. I really laid into one of them, this poor girl. She had thought it was the safest thing to do. Apparently Colin liked the girl from the Mildmay and she was going to pop in on a daily basis, but he'd refused to have anyone from the Social Services who were meant to be with him at night.

By this time my eldest sister and brother-in-law had arrived. The Social Services had gone into panic mode and they arrived back with the Area Manager to find out what the situation was. What they'd decided to do was that if Colin still didn't agree to have someone there twenty-four hours a day they would Section him and force him into hospital. That was something none of us wanted, none of us wanted him forced into hospital against his will.

So there we all were, Mum, my sister and her husband, Sean from the Mildmay, the Social Services, Sarah and me and suddenly Colin started talking absolute gibberish. It was as if his brain had slipped out of gear. We couldn't believe it was happening – I thought he was going to die right there in front of us. Then he suddenly said he'd agree to the twenty-four-hour care.

The next problem was that although he was still confused he had this enormous amount of anger which he channelled at Mum. She couldn't do anything right. He was hateful and said the most horrible things to her. She became more and more upset. We think it was because he really wanted to be at home with his mum, and that just wasn't on – she was sixty-eight, she'd got narrow stairs and you couldn't possibly get someone disabled up them. There was just no way she could have coped. The team from the Mildmay couldn't have gone that far out, and there wasn't any support around Enfield, nothing at all. It wasn't an option to consider and Colin felt quite bitter about it.

He was at home in his flat for a fortnight. Tower Hamlets were absolutely brilliant, they kept up the twenty-four-hour care, and the Mildmay said they would take him in any time, if we could persuade him to go.

We wanted to take Colin to the Mildmay for an afternoon visit, just so he could see the place. He'd managed to put his bath in the flat out of action. We don't know exactly what happened but he'd tried to re-pot all his plants in the bath, and the bath was totally blocked up. His carers tried to get someone in from the Council to fix the bath, but when they came round to try and unblock the hole they made too much noise and Colin sent them away! So we thought we could take him down to the Mildmay just to have a bath.

When Colin first faced up the fact of having AIDS, he sort of broke down and said, "I don't want to die," but from that time on he just seemed so confused, he just wanted to block everything out. So he definitely didn't want to go into the Mildmay, but after several days when my brother-in-law and I talked about it to him he agreed to go in for a visit.

When we took him in for the bath everyone was brilliant. From the very first moment we arrived, when the cleaning lady came up and took his hand, they just seemed so special. They showed Colin round one of the wards and asked him if he was hungry. It was mid-afternoon and everyone had already eaten, but they got him some dinner. Then he said he'd like a beer, which they managed to find for him – he didn't drink it, but it was a way of asserting himself.

The Mildmay were very keen to take him because they thought they could do so much more for him there than in the community. Colin liked the Mildmay. It was a bright, friendly place which seemed so removed from a hospital environment. So we finally made arrangements for him to go in on Good Friday, which was two weeks after he'd come out of hospital. We knew that long-term the Social Services couldn't keep up the care – they'd been absolutely brilliant for the two weeks, but it was a lot of money and resources to be tied up.

The phone never stopped ringing in this house because everyone rang here to find out what was happening. It was important that the others were kept in touch. Colin did look on me as the one who would sort him out if he needed it, and of course that did lead to tension. My sister and her husband were very supportive, we'd all got on well and we shared things. They did more than their fair share.

Once in the Mildmay we were amazed – first of all we were told that Colin only had a couple of weeks to live, and we conditioned ourselves to that. And then he picked up, he actually began walking again. We really didn't know where we were. We didn't think it was going to be that long but surprisingly it was; he was in the Mildmay for six months. Colin had two major problems, one was his legs and the other was the confusion. The doctors were trying to find out what the problem was. He was the first patient they'd had in there where the brain had been affected first. One of Colin's great fears was that he would lose his sight, but he never did. He was still on AZT when he went in and I was still convinced that the AZT was having a detrimental effect and after they reduced the dose he really picked up. My sister came over then from South Africa. That was another thing, the dilemma about should she come, should she not? We felt after he'd gone into the Mildmay that she should come over, but we didn't know whether he'd still be alive by the time she arrived. We'd given her this picture of gloom and doom, and when she arrived there was Colin, up and walking about with the aid of a Zimmer frame, sitting in the Mildmay eating his lunch.

Another difficulty was that you never knew with Colin whether it was him being bolshy or whether it was the condition, so you never knew how to behave with him. He got so incredibly demanding, always ringing on his buzzer for the nurses. Once he rang the bell and asked the nurse to clean his glasses for him! You'd say to him, "Look there are other people in here who are iller than you, who need the nurses more," and we'd try and talk him through it, but ten minutes later he'd ring again.

We found in the end we had to be quite hard with him, and say he couldn't go home for the weekend and stay with Mum or whatever it was. He got quite like a child, he seemed to need those parameters, and once he knew he couldn't push you any further he'd be all right. We'd go and visit and he'd be awful to us, and when we'd get up and say, "Look there's no point in us being here," he'd suddenly behave himself. But it was hard to find the courage to do that.

The other thing was he didn't seem to have any limitations any more on what he said or did. There was an occasion when he was in the foyer and he was on the telephone describing in a very loud voice how the nurse had to rub cream on to his willy because he had sores there, and all round him were these nice people visiting the Mildmay to see whether it would be a suitable place for their relatives!

He always wanted to be where he wasn't. Although he thought the Mildmay was wonderful, he'd suddenly want to go back to his flat, or to Mum's. He'd tell Mum he was getting a taxi and coming over. He was constantly baiting her till she got paranoid about it and thought that every car that drew up outside was him.

There's a noticeboard at the Mildmay, and there was a card advertising chauffeur-driven Rolls-Royces. So one day he got on the phone and ordered one, and no one knew that he'd done it until the car turned up at the front door and one of the nurses had to go down and explain it away. After that he was banned from using the phone without asking permission first. The other thing was that his ring had got too tight, because his finger had swollen. One of the volunteers was asked to arrange with a jeweller to take him there and get the ring cut off. The next day two fire engines turned up! The volunteer had rung up the fire brigade and asked if there was anyone who could come and cut the ring off, so when they were passing on some sort of exercise they all came in, all these burly firemen, to cut Colin's ring off!

Colin drove everyone completely mad, but he became quite a character in there. There were definitely some funny times. You can't say too much in praise of the Mildmay – some people think it's all religion, because of it being a Mission Hospital, but it's not. Religion's there is you want it but it's not thrust upon you. And it's a good place for families and partners, because they take the families in as much as the patient, the care of everybody is important to them.

There were weekly meetings and I'd go along and talk about what the best thing was to do for Colin, and we agreed that if he was well enough he could go home to Mum's at weekends. It was a lovely summer, so we could have barbeques and the whole family would come over.

His birthday was in the July and the whole family were at the Mildmay together, so we all sat down and worked out a visiting rota. That meant that Colin had at least one visitor every day during the week. At weekends we arranged it so that each member of the family took it in turns to be with him for the whole day. We'd either take him out to places like Greenwich or Rochester, or he would go home to Mum for the day. It was very important to him that there was always someone around.

SARAH

Colin came out every weekend right up until the week before he died. He got thinner and thinner and was wasting away, but he got up and dressed every day until the day before he died. He'd drive the nurses mad because he needed help to get out of bed, but six o'clock in the morning he'd want to get up. He never stayed in bed, he was obsessed with not being in bed.

We were popping in and out to see him and he was always pleased to see us even if it wasn't our turn. We were also trying to sort the flat out. The Council wasn't prepared to keep it on indefinitely, and we knew he'd never go back there but we couldn't tell him that.

He had a lot of plants there, and we suggested that we should bring them to the Mildmay. When we arrived with them on that Saturday he was suddenly quite poorly. He didn't seem to know quite what was going on. When we left that night we spoke to the nurses and they were thinking of upping the medication. We asked them to let us know if anything happened. It was our day on the Sunday, and he was too ill to come home. In fact that morning he hadn't wanted to get out of bed. So we phoned Mum in case she wanted to come in.

I think it's a myth that everyone goes through a great goodbye. People have this idea that with a terminal illness you have these heartfelt goodbyes, but it's not like that at all, and when the end comes it's just as big a shock. Although you think you're prepared for it, you never are.

PAUL

The next day Colin was sort of half with it and half not and he kept asking where he was. By this time, for the last couple of days, he was on morphine. Graeme, who's one of the volunteers at the Mildmay, was there. Colin had been away with Graeme on a week's holiday in Bournemouth. They stayed with a wonderful woman who takes in AIDS patients and after that Graeme had become like one of the family. He used to do a half day a week, and when it came to the end it happened that Graeme was there with me and my brother-in-law; my sister had just gone out. It was a very peaceful end, he just slipped away.

Colin had been a difficult patient, mainly because of the way the virus had affected his brain, and also because of his anger about having AIDS. On the other hand, he was also incredibly brave. He was confined to a wheelchair for over five months and lost a lot of weight which caused pressure sores in lots of places which were very difficult to treat. The nurses said it must have been extremely painful. He also had a permanent catheter, which caused several infections and again must have been very painful at times. But he never complained about the pain he was in or moaned about any treatment he was given, however uncomfortable it may have been. If anyone asked him how he was, whether it was a doctor, a friend, or family, he would always say, "Fine, thanks."

Colin never gave in to AIDS, and he fought with great courage right to the end. Sadly will power isn't enough to change the fate of AIDS sufferers, because I am sure if it was enough Colin would still be with us.

Colin often used to say "How much longer have I got?" which of course we couldn't answer. But then he'd never push it, he didn't want to discuss it and never talked about his funeral. We had a cremation locally. The word seemed to have got around and a few of his friends came, although he had lost touch with a lot of his friends. He'd had a buddy at the Mildmay. It was funny when she started because the first thing he asked her was if she had a car and, if so, could she take him over to his mum's! That was what he wanted from a buddy. She came to the funeral, and so did the

76

nurses from the Mildmay, several of the other staff, and Graeme. The Chaplain from the Mildmay took the service.

During Colin's illness we all thought carefully about who we told. We didn't tell those colleagues at work whom we thought might be horrified by it. In 1990 when this was all happening people were not quite so understanding about AIDS. I think things are better now, but there is still a lot of fear and prejudice around mainly due to people's ignorance. Mum found it terribly difficult – she didn't even want her own mother, who was still alive, to know. When she phoned up work she never said what the illness was and I think they think Colin died of cancer. I think that's what most mothers tell people if they are working with them. I think she also found it very hard to cope with him being gay.

The Mildmay was just so brilliant we wanted to put something back. Some months afterwards we went to the memorial service. These are held every six months, and the partners, family and friends of all those who have died during those six months are invited to come back. It's a moving service. All the names of those who have died are entered into a memorial book. We all went to that en masse, all the family. After that we did a ten-week course with them, one evening a week, to do voluntary work. You get to meet a lot of people from all walks of life, and all ages. We don't necessarily do an evening but we help out with driving which is something we can do together, which suits us, and we drive people home or to hospital, or we help out at events like the memorial services, making tea and things.

When you go through something like Colin's illness, you've got a lot of emotional pressures which you're not really aware of at the time because you've got all the day-to-day things to worry about. Suddenly when it's all over, you go through all the things you could have done or didn't do, the things you wanted to say and didn't, or the things you could have changed. You look at yourself, you analyse your whole life. Things that seemed important before this happened now seem quite meaningless, we've changed our attitude totally. Helping out at the Mildmay is part of that – keeping in touch with people at the Mildmay is important to us.

It's only when something like this happens that you realise that some of the things politicians go on about are meaningless. The important thing at the end of the day is the community, looking after the sick, the elderly, the blind, and in most areas they're just forgotten, just nuisances. But on the other side there are all the people at places like the Mildmay, all the buddies, the staff, the volunteers, they're just such genuine people. There's a lot of good out there.

ROBERT

I come from a farming family in Sussex and I've a brother and sister, both younger than me. My parents divorced when I was eight and I've rather lost touch with my father. So he doesn't know I'm ill. My mother, brother and sister have always known that I was gay and they've always been fantastic about that.

When I first got ill I told my mother exactly what was going on. I had been feeling lousy for a while with what I thought was flu and it kept getting worse. My brother-in-law is a hospital doctor and my sister brought him to see me, and he thought I had pneumonia. I'd been to the casualty department at St George's Tooting, in London, and they'd sent me home and told me to stop being so stupid. I discovered later that my brother-in-law had realised exactly what was the matter with me but he didn't want to be the one in the family to put up the alarm signals and begin a big emotional drama. He just thought I should get some professional help as soon as possible.

A couple of days later things got very bad and I suddenly couldn't get out of bed. My sister came round one evening and she called an ambulance to take me to hospital. When I got there I was terrified because I had suspected that this was AIDS pneumonia. I had a parrot in those days which had just had psittacosis, a form of pneumonia, so I convinced the hospital that I had psittacosis! I didn't let on about being gay or anything which was really very silly looking back, but I guess I was just very scared.

They shoved me on an antibiotic for psittacosis, which didn't of course do anything for the PCP! So for ten days I didn't get any better. After a while as I got worse I didn't know what was happening. I was in a general ward and I was unconscious for several days.

My partner Nick was in America. He'd been ringing the hospital every day and in the end he insisted that they tested me for HIV. I remember that when they came and told me the result I felt an overpowering sense of relief. It was a most extraordinary feeling and I've heard other people say the same thing. It was the end of seven years of worry – day by day worry of will this happen to me? How will I cope? How will the family cope?

I remember that evening. I'd been on different antibiotics for about twenty-four hours and I was just beginning to feel a bit better. Nick was with me when they told us and after the doctor left we both cried. It was really weird; I could tell that both of us felt we should cry but neither of us really wanted to.

Then Nick had an HIV test and it was positive. They did a T-cell count on him and his count came back at ten, when it should be a thousand. In any other country except Britain you're classed as having AIDS if the count's below two hundred, but in Britain you have to have had an illness. So there we were with him effectively in the AIDS group too.

In my own mind I'm sure how I got it. I went to work in America for a while, from 1979 until the mid-eighties, and of course AIDS was happening there in the early eighties. I had unprotected sex with various people. One of them was quite close to me and he died of AIDS in about 1984. In my own mind I've always been fairly convinced that it was him. I quite often think about him but with no resentment.

In about 1984 both Nick and I had been on holiday, and I felt lousy, as if I had flu. When you are infected with the virus, the virus is in the blood stream for about three months in a free state, and it doesn't create an antibody. And then at some stage after about three months it enters the body in a new kind of way and there's an antibody response. At that moment many people have symptoms that are very close to AIDS – night sweats, tiredness and enlarged glands, which all subside after a few months. People may think they've got glandular fever, or something like that, but it's now a recognised thing that you get these symptoms and an HIV test at that stage will be positive.

I had night sweats and someone said I should go and see a particular doctor in Harley Street. I realised when I was in his consulting room that he thought I had AIDS, but in those days very few people knew anything about the illness. Yes, OK, I had an enlarged spleen, an enlarged liver and swollen glands – but I was virtually classified dead ten minutes after I landed up in his waiting-room! He said he wanted me to go into St Mary's that same afternoon, but I said I couldn't cope with that. I just wasn't prepared suddenly to land up on a ward and so I didn't go. Now I realise that he was terribly excited to have found an AIDS patient but he didn't tell me that I had AIDS, and if he had I probably wouldn't have believed him.

It was then that Nick and I started going to a homeopath in the West End. I didn't like him very much but he said to me, "You have not got AIDS!" and of course the relief was terrific. But then began the seven years of wondering.

My mother visited me a lot when I went into hospital with the PCP and she knew that they were going to do the HIV test. In the evening I phoned her from the sister's office to tell her that they'd confirmed I had AIDS. That was a fantastic moment for me, for both of us. She just said to me, "Darling, you know I love you and I'll love you whatever, and this makes no difference to that. We're going to get through this together." I knew that telling her wouldn't be any kind of problem beyond being sad.

When I was in hospital I was offered counselling – there were Peter and Ralph and they used to creep in to talk to us. One of them was a real creeper and what Nick calls a "nodder" so that whenever we said anything he would nod in deep understanding! Nick and I kept getting the giggles when they came to talk to us and I think after a few days they realised that this was not very productive!

All my friends came in to see me and my brother and sister. The only person in the family we haven't told about my illness is my grandmother, whom I'm very fond of and who's a wonderful lady. She knows I'm gay and she's absolutely fantastic about that. She always sends letters to "My darlings Robert and Nick . . ." In fact we have decided to talk to her this Easter and tell her. Even though she's elderly, her mind is completely intact, so why shouldn't she know? I feel very strongly that it's wrong not to tell her, I feel I'm being deceitful.

My family has been wonderful. I realise I'm incredibly lucky – unlike Nick, whose family to this day do not know that he's gay or that he has AIDS, and this is three years on. They don't want to know – he sees them a lot and he's tried to tell them. He works in television and he made a very explicit film drama about a boy who goes home to tell his parents he's gay. He gave his parents a tape of this before it went out and said, "Look, this is a really personal thing that I've done here, please watch it." There was silence for a few days and then they phoned. His father came on to the phone and said that he did not consider this subject fit subject matter for television. He then said, "Nick, I have to tell you that I probably know a great deal more about homosexuality than you ever will – I was in the army and the desert, and in the desert I saw the depths of depravity to which men can sink. I'll hand you over to your mother."

His mother came on the line and said, "Nick, all I can say is that I hope that no child of mine would ever be so cruel as to come home and tell me that kind of filth." So after that we've rather given up.

When I came out of hospital I decided to spend a couple of weeks with my mum, just to be there. I had talked to her about telling the people she knew socially what was wrong with me. I thought, and she had agreed, that I didn't want it hidden from anybody. I felt I never wanted to feel that I couldn't say something. I also felt that it was important for people to meet people with AIDS to see that they were fairly normal. She lives very much in the middle-class environment on the outskirts of Tunbridge Wells, it's all rather *The Archers*.

To my amazement, and what I thought was fantastically brave, she had already told quite a few of her friends. She's a teacher in special education and she had decided not to tell anyone at the school because she was afraid that parents would react badly because of their own children. But we went to tea with this local family we've known for years. Hugh, the father, is a nice man but in the past I'd never done anything more than shake his hand – it was only in the last few years I'd even managed to call him Hugh and not Mr! But when we arrived he came up to me and hugged and kissed me. I remember being absolutely knocked out by that and thinking what a generous and brave thing it was to do.

My mother has been a bit selective about who she's told. She was talking the other day about telling a couple more friends and I've encouraged her to because so far nobody's been anything but supportive. I think you have to risk telling people. When they think about AIDS in the abstract they probably think about it with horror. But when a friend – someone you're fond of – tells you that someone close to them has AIDS I think people react differently, and they care.

I'd decided that I would go on to AZT. At that time the hospital was recommending 800 milligrams a day and I decided to take 400 milligrams. A year ago I stopped taking it although I hadn't had any side effects at all – none of the things I'd heard about such as sickness or headaches. But a year ago they suddenly told me that one of my white blood cell counts was quite low and they thought it might well be because of the AZT. It was at exactly the same time as I got KS. They'd done the blood count because of the KS, because sometimes when there's a new infection it's because of a low cell count. I thought it was crazy – on the one hand they were telling me I was taking AZT to stop me getting all these problems, but it was the AZT that was causing me the problems at the same time! So for the last year I've only taken Pentamidine once a month. It's an inhalation and I've got an air pump.

When I left my mother's I came back here, to the house I share with Nick and a Dutch friend Gijs. I remember being absolutely obsessed with it being filthy and thinking that I was going to catch everything in this house, from all these dogs and cats and the parrot. I was very scared. I really thought I wouldn't live for more than a couple of months and that I'd be back in hospital with some other ghastly thing.

After my convalescence we entered this strange new territory of wondering and waiting. Over the first couple of months there were quite a lot of phone calls – how are you and things – and then life sort of returned to normal.

Once you've got AIDS there's a kind of understanding of how

your life is going to go. But with HIV it's difficult. Gijs is HIV positive and I think he finds it all much more difficult to cope with. He was a teacher in Holland and I think he's made some very good decisions – his real passion in life is music and he suddenly applied for and got on to a four-year course at music college. He wants to be a performer and I know he sometimes thinks that the irony will be that he'll do his four-year course, and then he'll be ill.

Initially I went to the clinic once a month. They have these community nurses and we were assigned one who came to visit the house. I think I needed a lot of reassurance at first, but I carried on working as a journalist. I even went back to playing squash and to swimming, and feeling as if I hadn't been ill at all.

I got PCP again last November and the hospital had terrible trouble diagnosing it. They kept giving me X-rays and the X-rays kept showing this massive chest infection but I was walking around feeling fine. They did eventually do a bronchoscopy and that time I took the antibiotics orally at home.

I only stopped working last Christmas, really because I was increasingly not enjoying writing articles about things I didn't really care about. I just wasn't getting a great deal of pleasure out of it. I was also spending more and more time having to go to hospital. The KS involved chemo and radiotherapy and that means huge numbers of visits to the hospital. Of course I could be writing this afternoon but sometimes the last thing I want to do after a morning of fighting depression as you lie on those radiotherapy beds is sit down and clock into writing.

I've claimed all the benefits I'm entitled to and I can't tell you how fantastically lucky I've been. I was up-to-date with all my stamps so I've got income support and mobility allowance. They've been very generous to me. There's my new Peugeot car outside – very often people don't know they may be entitled to that. If you receive the higher rate of mobility allowance, which anybody with AIDS automatically does, you're entitled to join the Motability scheme.

What you do is you swop your £31 a week, your mobility allowance from the DSS, for the car. I went to my local Peugeot dealer and said this would be a Motability scheme. He said, good, that'll be easy! Two weeks later I drove this car out of the dealers.

They give you free road tax, free insurance, full AA membership free, all your garage bills and any replacement tyres and wind-screens free. The other great thing is that the insurance covers one other person to drive as well.

When I got ill I refused to go back to the homeopathic quack we'd gone to but I'd heard about a homeopath called Mike Strange, in Clapham, and I went to see him. I have found him fantastic. I think I do have quite good faith in homeopathy, though I am a bit of a doubting Thomas at times. I'll go for a month or two thinking it's brilliant, and then for a couple of months I'll think it's rubbish. The trouble is I love drinking coffee and all the things you're not meant to do! I think Mike is a good homeopath but his real skill is that you can walk in there feeling fed up and walk out feeling fantastic, really lifted. He gives you tremendous confidence and reassurance. It must be so exhausting to do it but he's been really good. There are lots of packets of little white pills around the place which I keep forgetting to take.

I decided when I got ill that I wasn't going to be a passive patient. The hospital must sometimes hate Nick and I when we march into the clinic slapping down articles from the *Lancet*, or new information about treatments under trial in the United States, demanding to know why we're not on this, that or the other.

I sometimes see a wry smile on the face of my consultant as I struggle to talk on equal terms about the significance of blood test results and drug therapies. But I do this because I think it's so important that as a patient I remain in control of the decisions made about me. The great thing about St George's Hospital is that they have allowed me to do this, there's no "Yes, Doctor, No Doctor". If I think the doctor is wrong I tell him. The deal we have is that Mark, my consultant, and his team give me the information that allows me to make the decision.

Recently I've had to make a decision about chemotherapy. I have a form of cancer common in AIDS and it's spread to my lungs. My doctors told me I could try systemic chemotherapy using a drug called Bleomycine. We agreed that before making a decision I would spend a couple of weeks thinking about it, researching everything I could on the side effects and effectiveness of the treatment. When I first got ill with AIDS a senior pharmacist came up to see me on the ward and gave me her bleep number so that if I had any query about any drug I could ask for more information. This has been invaluable. So after a couple of weeks of intense research into Bleomycine, phoning other hospitals and AIDS organisations such as the Terrence Higgins Trust, I was able to decide that this was not a treatment I wanted for myself and that I would rather take my chances with no treatment at all.

Another great thing about St Georges is that they will, if you ask them, withhold all treatment while you're on the ward so that a homeopath or other alternative practitioner can come in and treat you. But of course when I had PCP I just wanted to be better.

I've talked to some of the chemists who make AZT and I know that there is a feeling there that AZT may not be the wonder drug it was cracked up to be. And there's increasing evidence from the United States to support this. The AZT trials are all so dodgy when you look at them and the results are dodgy too. We know it's a fantastically toxic drug to take and I simply don't think there's evidence that it prolongs life. Sure, since AZT became available people do live much longer but at the same time doctors learnt how to cure and prevent the infections, such as PCP that had been causing the early deaths of so many. AZT took the credit but I have serious doubts about whether or not it should.

There is no doubt that you turn yourself into an expert very quickly and it's easy to do that. There's a fantastic amount of information available. I have a filing cabinet upstairs and there's a whole section of it called AIDS. There's information on everything. Body Positive are always publishing things and a friend in New York sends me all the latest stuff. I talk to the doctors a lot about this and perhaps they find it unnerving that a patient should want such control over their treatment. Certainly the relationship between me and my doctors is more that of a professional friend, with them supplying the information and me making the decisions.

Recently Nick's father was in Guy's Hospital having a heart operation and I remember Nick getting the shock of his life, because the doctors were all Mr So and So. When he asked his father when he was coming home it was "Oh, not till Mr So and So says it's all right." "And why are you taking these tablets?"

"Because they've just given them to me." He said it was like walking back into the last century.

I call my consultant Mark and tease him and tell him he hasn't a clue what he's talking about! I challenge him and tell him I'm not happy and I'm going off to talk to other experts about things. After you've had AIDS for three years, you are an expert – I can read blood results now as well as any doctor!

I think the reason why patients are able to behave like this is because the doctors can't offer any hope. They can offer help but not hope. So unlike a cancer patient who can be forced down a certain road because of the chance of the cure at the end of it, I can turn round and say, "No, you have not yet saved anybody, I'm going to do it my way", and I think that makes the doctors feel very powerless. My aunt died of cancer a few years ago and all the time I felt she was being pushed into all these horrendous drug treatments because there was always this faint hope that she might get well again. As a result nobody was allowed to think about death in the way that death is ever-present with AIDS. Unlike cancer, it's inevitable that you're going to die of AIDS. There is nobody around you can point to who has survived it.

After I got ill, I did have this very strong feeling that I wanted someone to talk to outside of family and friends, but I didn't know who or what. I kept thinking I didn't want a "counsellor" and I started to think a lot myself about what was going on. I decided that this illness might be destroying my body but I didn't think it was destroying me. And that was confusing because I had always thought of my body and me as the same and now I was saying they were separate.

I talked to my mother and she found me someone through a priest friend of hers. He is quite the most extraordinary guy I've ever met. He's extraordinary in that he's so ordinary. He was then the rector of St Botolph's in Aldgate. He arrived at this church twenty years ago, he looked around and saw this problem of the homeless in the City of London but there was nothing to help them. By the time he moved to a new job last year he had a full-time paid staff of forty-five, and 120 volunteers, nurses and doctors and dentists. There's a huge extension and the whole place runs on a million pound budget.

The first time I met him he came here to see me and I was so disappointed! I had expected some very dramatic character and in comes this ordinary looking vicar. Once a month for the last three years, we have spent an afternoon talking. Mostly we talk about things like boxing – it's not very structured! But I like to know he's there if I suddenly feel I need to talk. The first time I met him he asked me what sort of funeral I wanted, and I remember being terribly taken aback and thinking help! and I said to him hey, I'm still here! But he's very good at occasionally making you confront things, and I've grown very fond of him – I am about to ask him if he will conduct my funeral.

A year ago I told him that I was so sick of the world of journalism I want to do something else as well. He suggested I do some volunteer work at the St Botolph's Centre for the Homeless. To start with I was a bit dubious but it's now become an important part of my life. I cook lunch there every Tuesday and in the afternoon do a discussion group. The staff all know that I have AIDS and I was very pleased when they asked me if I would talk about AIDS at a training day.

The HIV thing is a small part of the life at St Botolph's but I am horrified to see how many homeless HIV people there are – lots of them are, or were, drug users. They get no emotional support and they're often people whose lives have become so disorganised they will turn up at a hospital casualty rather than a clinic. They're not good at making or keeping appointments and they often don't take their medication, or they lose it.

For me the work has been wonderful – it's one day a week, so it's not the bulk of my time and I find some of the issues surrounding homelessness fascinating. Eighty per cent of people on the street are there with mental health problems. When you talk to them you find they've all been in hospital at some time or another.

About a year ago I went home to Mum for the weekend and she and I had this terrible row because I told her that I felt the whole family should be engaged in some sort of counselling. She was furious with me and didn't want this at all. I think she was angry because she didn't want the whole family to start talking about me dying. Sometimes I feel concerned because we could find ourselves in a situation where things have suddenly turned rather nasty, for the worse, and then they'll be dealing with it all in a crisis. I do tell my mother everything that's happening medically. She knows that at the moment I'm having radiotherapy and chemo and during this week I've talked to her once or twice. I don't want to keep any secrets from her. But we are very secretive about how we each feel. We've moved from being very open about our feelings – I'd always talked to her about my relationships or whatever in the past but I find it hard now to talk about those things now because I can feel both of us getting tenser and tenser as we get closer to the real subject.

On crisis days we do have these circular phone conversations. I'll phone my mother to say "They think I've got PCP again." She'll say, "Darling, I am sorry. Are you all right?" And I say "Yes, actually, I seem to be quite well at the moment, I'll be fine." "Good, good, that all sounds very positive." I ask her "Are you feeling all right about it?" and she'll say, "Yes, yes fine" and within seconds she's on the phone to my brother, "Oh God, he's got PCP, do you think I should go to London?" Then my brother will phone me and say, "She's been on the phone, she's in floods of tears . . .!" Then I wonder whether I should go and see her. A lot of that goes on.

It's hard to talk to Mum about it because she's going to lose her eldest son and that's always going to be terribly difficult to talk about, and I'm sure she doesn't want to face it. I'm not sure also what there is to be talked about.

I sometimes feel I want to say "I'm sorry – I'm sorry I'm doing this to you, to the family". I can say it easily to others, but if she was sitting here she and I would be in floods of tears. I think my over-riding feeling about it is that this is going totally to destroy the rest of my mother's life. She's sixty and if she lives for another twenty years, this is never going to go away. And nothing would give me greater pleasure than to die knowing that she was feeling that we had resolved some of these things between us. I don't think Mum has any idea of what's coming in terms of the disabilities – I mean I've seen guys who are quite disabled and ill for a year or so, and that's the scary one.

My sister asked her husband what the future might be and I know she stopped him after about a minute. She couldn't take it.

One of the things about AIDS is that you usually have time to prepare yourself for dying; you prepare the family for it; make the appropriate arrangements and make sure that nothing's left in a muddle. I think that's a positive thing.

I was talking to a friend whose partner died about eighteen months ago and I said to him, "You don't seem to have grieved in the way I thought you would." He said, "By the time he died I had poured out so much emotion and invested so much into this thing that it was strange – obviously I think about him every day but I can do it with a sense of relief in a way."

Nick and I do have this sense that where our friends are concerned we have to put on this incredibly brave face. Lots of our friends are gay and lots of them are worried about or have HIV. We have somehow got into this routine of belittling AIDS – you know, it's really not that bad, the radiotherapy isn't too bad. It's so easy to become an AIDS bore so I'm quite careful if I'm going to dinner with people not to talk about it. I do have one or two friends who I talk to privately about having AIDS, but that's probably more to do with my concern for Nick than to do with me. I've got two other friends who I can see are in that stage of moving from just being HIV to having AIDS. Both have got skin rashes, and looking back I know that's how it all started with us. One of them said to me the other day, "Rob, I've got this rash, what do you think?" I said, "Yes, it could be HIV-related, then again it might not be. Everyone gets rashes." But I was thinking to myself that it was how it had started with me – rashes that never quite went away – and looking at my friend's rash I felt incredibly sad whilst trying to sound reassuring. We have to be made to feel we can cope, somehow, but sometimes it's a fragile kind of coping.

I have a friend at the moment who's very ill. I look at him and think he's got such dignity. He seems to cope so amazingly well with things like the dentist, his hair, buying new clothes or just being around publicly. He seemed to me to do it with such poise and dignity, and I find that so encouraging. A lot of the time life must be such a struggle but he has avoided becoming a bag of illness. He's remained Michael and remained interested and involved in the world around him. There are people who just give in at some point and become ill, ill, ill, and then there are others like Michael who can't deny that they're ill but have decided that it's not the focus of their life, that they're still going to be somebody.

We had a dinner party not long ago and there were thirteen people whom we knew quite well, some very well. Suddenly someone asked "Who round this table knows that they're HIV positive?" To our absolute disbelief, everyone put their hands up. So we're not at all isolated but I think there is a down side to the familiarity. You're rather encouraged to belittle your own illness.

I'm always astonished when heterosexuals don't take AIDS seriously. When I'd been ill for about a year, my brother phoned me very very upset one day. A few days before he'd gone to visit a girl whom he was having an affair with who was still living with her ex-boyfriend who was having an affair of his own. When my brother visited her, the ex-boyfriend was not at all well. He had flu and was so breathless that my brother said all he could think of was me when I had PCP pneumonia. He told this guy that he should get attention quite quickly. He was sent to hospital and put on a certain ward in the hospital which was the AIDS ward. My brother then said he'd been having unprotected sex with this girl for six months and she'd been having unprotected sex with her ex-boyfriend for seven years. They all went and had the HIV test and by some sheer luck they were all negative. That was about a year ago and I went with him to get the results of the test. I remember his relief and the tears of remorse.

Just last week he told me that his current girl friend was in hospital because she had tingling and numbness in her hands. Without thinking I said, "Oh yes, that's another AIDS symptom!" and he went absolutely cold on me. In fact she wasn't on the AIDS ward but he looked so stricken that I asked him why he was so worried? And then it came out that he was having unprotected sex with her. I said, "For heavens sake, with me, your past experience, what the hell were you doing? Why don't you use condoms?" And he said he didn't like them! We talked about it and I realised that it's so outside the culture of that heterosexual world that even when someone comes as close to AIDS as my brother had done, they still cannot believe it exists or might happen to them.

Meanwhile my partner Nick is amazing – he has the energy he's always had and he's working very hard. He has skin problems and sometimes they've been quite severe, causing quite nasty temperatures. He keeps testing positive to CMV and when this happens the hospital phone up to alert us which generates a horrible feeling of crisis. CMV is something to avoid because it can make you blind and you have to start a horrendous drug regime. But so far every time they have re-tested Nick the CMV has returned to negative. Sometimes looking up all these drugs and knowing all about them is not necessarily such a good idea. Once when they wanted to put Nick on a drip I read the literature on a particular drug and it said it shouldn't be given to anyone unless the patient isn't expected to live for more than twelve months! Scary. So Nick refused the drug but he asked them to keep testing him for CMV. So one week he tests positive and the next week negative and they don't know why. I don't think it's ever happened like this before. He goes and has his eyes looked at regularly and so far they're fine.

Nick and I do have sex outside our relationship. It's something I think a great deal about and I find very complicated. We have never had a truly monogamous relationship. He travels abroad quite a lot and sometimes there are long periods when he's away. During those times sometimes I've mucked about and sometimes he's mucked around. Since I've been ill I've been to bed with a number of people whom I've not told that I was HIV and I would also claim that on those occasions I've been safe. Nick would say exactly the same. I have also been to bed with people and told them I was HIV positive. No one has ever walked out the door. Why I don't always tell people I don't know. It's partly fear.

Nick still sleeps around occasionally. The other day there was somebody he wanted to sleep with and I asked him whether he was going to tell them that he was HIV positive and he said he didn't know. I think that as they got into bed he told him and the person was so bloody understanding that he couldn't do it anyway!

Most of my gay friends will say that if they go to a bar they wouldn't expect someone who was HIV positive to tell them because it's part of our culture that it's your responsibility to be safe to yourself. Morally I do find this difficult. I think it is wrong not to tell people you're HIV positive. I think it's a real problem in gay relationships – you meet someone, you sleep with them a couple of times and then you begin to get fond of them and you're in this terrible position of having deceived them. It goes without saying that I would never have sex without taking precautions.

I've thought a lot about dying. I remember suddenly saying to Mike Strange in a totally extravagant moment, "Right, I feel really confident about dying! I've sorted this out!" I could see him saying to himself, stupid boy! But I do feel confident about dying. The fear is about the practical side. I worry that Nick won't be able to cope with me being ill.

The other evening we had the most terrible dinner party of our lives. I'd spent the whole day having chemotherapy. They'd injected my eye so that it was like a golf ball and I was in a huge amount of pain. I staggered to Sainsbury's, feeling like death, and shopped for the ten people I'd invited. There was a huge amount of shopping and I was in a rage because, as usual, Nick had gone off to work. By the time everyone arrived I'd hit the bottle and the pheasants were all burning. A friend I'm very fond of and his wife came and he was drunk too. Suddenly he started saying "I've never been able to say this before but I just want you to know how I feel, how sad I feel that you're ill, how much I love you" . . . etc., and I was sitting there with this eye swollen up and looking dreadful. In the end I couldn't cope with it at all so I said I was going to bed. Then Nick came up and we were both upstairs in floods of tears. Finally he managed to get himself downstairs and went into the dining-room, and there they all were looking at him and he cried again.

One of our friends had brought along his latest lad – he was very young, a landscape gardener, and Nick suddenly turned on him with his eyes streaming with tears and shouted at him, "And what the hell do you do about safe sex? When did you last use a condom, and how dare you just pick people up in pubs and bars!" This poor lad just sat there, completely gob-smacked, and everyone just sort of packed up and went home! Ghastly.

If I ever feel the need to be in bed for a couple of days, or if it was increasingly difficult for me to get downstairs and make myself some lunch, I just think the stresses between us are going to become so enormous. After that awful dinner party my eye was so swollen and sore I decided I would spend the day in bed, and I could see Nick having to try really hard not to say something – he managed not to say anything then but he did say to me later, "I do hope you're not going to give in!" And I did think to myself, when it gets bad, we're going to need some outside help here.

In the gay community it's interesting but you never hear the word AIDS used any more. It's always ILL, as if there's only one illness in the world. I suppose there really is only one illness for gay people under fifty. I think there is a siege mentality in the gay community where AIDS is concerned – it does feel like war where people are dropping off around you. But I have an elderly friend who's eighty something, and he said it was just like when he was a young man with TB, which was the same sort of long-drawn-out illness.

MELANIE

When I was told of the diagnosis it all seemed so unreal. I couldn't believe it all. I'm told I was very calm but all I felt was sheer terror. There was also the sense of, "My God I want to rush out and tell someone." But then a voice at the back of my mind said, hang on – you can't say lightly to someone you're HIV and then pretend you never said it. Once it's said, that's it, it's told for ever. To begin with I didn't tell anyone, which was quite a strain. When I had to go the hospital for the tests and to get the result I took time off work – as far as my colleagues were concerned I was having a cervical smear. So when I looked upset after the diagnosis they assumed that the smear had been dodgy. I was very aware that the longer the deception went on the more complicated things would become. There was a real sense of isolation and fear – and that was because of people's ignorance about the disease. That's why I feel so strongly that we need to educate people.

I wasn't living with my family at the time, and we weren't terribly close, so I didn't tell them. We've never discussed it and now we don't have any contact at all. I've come to terms with that – I get my support from my circle of friends, not my family. I did try and tell my mum, indirectly, but I found it much easier to tell my friends than my mother. First of all I tried to prepare the ground but then the words just wouldn't come out. I ended up giving her a series of heavy hints – I was sure she got the message, but she steered away from it. Yes, she'd got the message but her message back was that she didn't want to discuss it so I gave up. I'm an only child so I felt I was very much alone. This thing was with me and I was going to have to deal with it myself and not with my family. I suppose it's because AIDS is to do with sex – my mother's generation doesn't discuss sex – and there was no way she was going to discuss sex or HIV with me.

I've got a veneer and I gain strength from my friends. But I still have moments when I regret not telling Mum, when I think I'd like to talk to her. But, sadly, it's too late for that.

I was terrified about telling the first person: but she was marvellous. There was no feeling of, help, we can't share the coffee cups. She was absolutely the same. We rarely talk about it now – there's no need to – she doesn't cosset me or wrap me in cotton wool, which makes me feel good. The only change in our relationship is that she takes more of an interest in me.

I can't understand why people are still so frightened about AIDS, I really do have a problem with that. Unless you have unprotected sex with someone who's HIV positive you really are unlikely to catch it. I'm very aware of a lot of prejudice. I do have one friend, a gay man, and when I told him I was HIV positive he couldn't bring himself to touch me. He has a quite unreasonable fear and it really does hurt for someone like that not to want to hug me.

I think there's a great potential to educate children from a young age. The big problem about talking to children is that you're going to have to talk about sex, and sex is the big taboo. No one is comfy with talking about it openly, it makes adults feel very uncomfortable.

AIDS is still being treated like TB was years ago and the time will come when AIDS will be treated just as TB is now. But for me things are not changing quickly enough.

Most of the women I know who are HIV are lucky with their families, and all have good and positive relationships. I have friends with AIDS whose children don't know the full extent of the illness – and I understand why they don't tell their children. They fear for the children, for what they may suffer from the prejudice they may encounter.

I'm very lucky to be in London, because of the huge HIV and AIDS support. Many people with HIV or AIDS gravitate to London, not to escape their families necessarily but to be anonymous. The problem then becomes that the services are overburdened. There are HIV services outside London but they're usually under used and I can understand why. It's the isolation and the feeling of the stigma attached to the disease. In London there is a lot of goodwill. I've felt much more comfortable since I moved to London and discovered what is available to me. I'm very involved with a support group at the London Lighthouse. I feel very safe, I can be very honest and open about being a woman living with HIV. I'm aware though that it's a false sense of security. Lots of people can't uproot and move to London and I'm lucky.

MARK *was bi-sexual, and was married to Karen. He worked as an office manager for a large firm of estate agents in London. Karen was and indeed still is a nurse. They lived in the East End of London. Mark died two years ago when he was 47.*

KAREN

When we married we both knew that Mark might test HIV positive at some later date. He could have been tested before we were married, but we had decided not to do that. So from the time we were married we both knew the risks, and we always used condoms – and don't believe people when they say they don't work!

We'd thrashed it all out before we got married, so we were always expecting it to happen, although we certainly didn't expect it to happen so quickly. That's what took both of us by surprise, that it could happen so quickly.

We'd been married over a year, about 16 months, when Mark discovered he had AIDS. He'd been very unwell for a week, with night sweats and a high temperature, and feeling really ill. Then one day he felt so ill that I got the doctor and he was transferred to the local hospital. They diagnosed the illness as pneumonia, possibly TB. In fact they didn't come back with a final and definite diagnosis. I suspected though that it might be AIDS, in fact we both did.

After some intensive treatment they suggested that we be counselled and then tested for HIV. He had the test two or three weeks after his illness was over. He'd had a relapse, after he'd been out of hospital for four weeks, and he'd been back at work about a week. That's when we started going to the Middlesex. We both went in for initial counselling prior to having the test. So then it was just a question of waiting for the inevitable, waiting for the actual result.

Mark had never been ill in his life – the only time he'd been in hospital was when he had his tonsils out as a child. So although he could have been HIV for quite some time, he'd never had a day's sickness. He was perfectly healthy, that's what the biggest shock was.

My initial feeling when he was diagnosed as having AIDS was first how long had he got? Then there was almost a feeling of relief that somehow now we knew and we could deal with it together. As a nurse I felt better now that we knew positively that he was ill. I found that easier to cope with than worrying all the time about when he would get ill.

Mark's main worry after the diagnosis was about losing his mental faculties – he was a man who loved conversation, reading books, listening to music, so that was his main fear – that and the fear of blindness. He was angry, I think, there was quite a lot of that, the "Why me" feelings. You go through those kind of stages,

96

and you get past them. But he was more terrified than angry, and terrified of the dying bit. Although we'd talked it through and worked it through, when he was feeling grotty and getting ill, it was the fear of dying and letting go which got to him.

I was never frightened of catching AIDS. I was frightened because I didn't know very much about it, and I do remember going to the doctor at the Middlesex and saying, you know I'm not too sure about this – what happens if he has a bath and I have a bath afterwards! I just didn't know anything about it at that stage. At the beginning, because I was so ignorant, I didn't even know if there were special precautions you should take with cups and saucers! And of course the answer is no – there are only certain ways you can catch AIDS – the main way being by sleeping with someone. But at the beginning I really didn't know much about the details of the physical transference of the disease.

One of the main problems is that because there are so many physical illnesses related to AIDS, you never know what you're going to get next, which makes it different from having for example cancer. When you get AIDS, you get pneumonia, herpes – you know about the standard things you might get. But they don't tell you about the terrifying diarrhoea, the stomach cramps, the general tiredness. So you're always living with the terrifying uncertainty – had he got cerebral CMV that day when he seemed a bit disorientated? That was the worst strain, not knowing how long he'd got, not knowing how the disease was going to progress.

As he went along with the various illnesses I did read up about the specific things, but we didn't try and find out about everything, or read up about everything. We just took it as it came, and we listened to the people around us.

He'd only just started his job in December, and he got ill in February. By the time he was better it was May. So he'd been off work for such a long time that I had to discuss his ill health with the directors of the firm. I didn't tell them what was wrong with him, I just told them he'd had pneumonia, with a relapse. There was no way they could keep him on, because obviously they were paying him for not being there. So at that stage in about May, he lost his job, which was fair enough.

He didn't try and get another job, because really of the nature of the illness and all the stress that's involved. Anyway we felt that we could manage financially with just me working on my reasonable whack of a salary. And we were picking up Income Support too, so we managed quite well.

Our initial feeling when we first found out Mark was HIV positive was only to tell the people close to us, my best friend, and his best friend. As time went on though the strain of my working, together with the demands of him being ill, made it impossible not to tell other people.

At work it began to get very difficult – I had to keep remembering every time when he was ill what I had told them last time – was he meant to be convalescing this week, or had I said that last week? That's why we told as many people as we could. We needed them to support us, and to know what was going on.

I don't know whether the neighbours had their suspicions, but I told them Mark had lung cancer – and then felt awful when one of them died from lung cancer! We just felt that we wouldn't be able to cope with the lack of understanding, and we were very frightened of being shunned just when we really were going to need their support. At Mark's funeral, I remember I had to whizz round the people who did know he had AIDS and ask them not to mention the cause of death, because of all the people there who didn't know.

You have no conception of time when these things are happening to you, and it's still difficult now when you look back, but after the first two bouts of pneumonia I think he was then all right for a couple of months.

Initially when I went off to work, he pottered about at home, doing the shopping, taking the dog out for a walk, resting and reading. There were periods when he went to the Mildmay for a week, or went to stay with his best friend for a week. And then we went away for a week with the dog, that sort of thing.

The good thing about my work was that when I got there, I'd go into automatic pilot. I just used to go in, I had a job to do, and I could just switch off from home and get absorbed in the job. At the time I didn't seem to get too tired, but looking back I was pretty knackered. I had a friend living with us for the last six months of his illness, so that was a great help. But looking back, when I think of everything I did, I was pretty tired.

By this time Mark was on AZT – he'd gone on to that after the second bout of pneumonia. That was good, it didn't seem to have any side effects. He didn't get very many illnesses – he had the pneumonia, he got some thrush in the oesophagus, and they treated that, but inbetween that AZT seemed to do him well. His blood always seemed to be OK, and he certainly never needed any blood transfusions. He used to go through stages when he lost his appetite quite a lot, and certainly didn't feel like eating, but all in all, knowing what I know now, he did pretty well.

He did have one bout of toxoplasmosis, in August. He rang me one morning at work at about ten o'clock and said that it had taken him about half an hour to remember my telephone number. He'd come downstairs because he wanted to go for a pee, and he actually hadn't quite made it. He'd managed to get into the toilet and couldn't find his way out, and was a bit unsure about where he was.

So that was it, I just left work and came home straightaway. I stayed with him all day and he seemed not too bad. He pottered about and I just did my usual bits and pieces. And then he came down to have something to eat, and halfway through the meal he suddenly stopped eating and said he felt most peculiar and went upstairs. When I went upstairs into the bedroom he wasn't quite sure who I was, and that was it.

It was frightening, I didn't know what it was, or even whether it was something to worry about. I'd rung the doctor in the day, and he'd said, see how he goes, and when I rang him the second time he said it was likely to be toxoplasmosis. So I called an ambulance and he went straight into the hospital, and the hospital confirmed the toxo diagnosis. The treatment took about ten days to two weeks. At the time it was terrifying. I spoke to the doctors at length and they reckoned it would be three to six months once the toxoplasmosis had set in, so it was pretty scary. I even phoned his sister in Australia and told her that I wasn't quite sure what was going on.

By that stage most people knew what was going on, although there were still one or two who didn't know, and there were some people I remember telling after the toxo, for various reasons. I didn't tell my aunt and uncle. They live nearby and I'm close to them. I put it to them that it was a brain secondary from the original cancer, which they knew he already had. It was to protect them. There was always a feeling of not wanting to put people in a position where they then have to choose whether or not to carry on seeing you or not. That probably doesn't make much sense when I say it now, but at the time it made a lot of sense. We just felt it was better left unsaid.

People were always making awful remarks – things like, well they deserve it – I suppose because AIDS is seen as a homosexual thing. At work, I'd notice comments like, "Don't sit on that chair, you know who sat on it last." There was a survey of nursing staff a few years back, and lots of them still believed you can catch it from the swimming pool. That sort of thing made me groan – when you're going through it yourself, that's the last thing you need. It made life very difficult – because I was very conscious that I needed people to sympathise with me, to have compassion for me, to know what I was going through.

That's why I went and got counselling. I met Sister Eva Heymann, who works at the Terrence Higgins Trust, through the Health Adviser at the Middlesex who asked whether I wanted to go to her and get some counselling. When I heard she was a nun, I thought she'd be in the black penguin suit, but of course she's not like that at all. I used to go to her every couple of weeks.

You need a safe place to go to express the things you're thinking, things you can't say to your friends. You get a nice objective view, you don't have to feel selfish about it. I always felt I could cope, and do everything on my own, but there were times of sheer desperation.

After a while I went whenever I felt I needed to. She was very important to me – because I could go and talk things through that I couldn't talk to my family and friends about. I needed the reassurance that everything I was feeling was quite normal. I used to love going – I found it very fulfilling, very useful and very comforting. There were things I couldn't discuss with my mum and sister – they were always there and very reassuring, but they didn't know quite what to say to me. So it seemed sensible to go outside the family circle, to people who are trained to ask the right sort of questions.

The uncertainty of the illness was what made me realise I had to look after myself as well as looking after Mark. I was getting very stressed, and I learnt that I had to allow myself to stand back because no one knew how long the diseases would last – he could have gone on for years. The difficulty about it all is trying to get some perspective of what your life used to be like before it.

One of the worst moments was when I walked out on him when he was in hospital. He was being bloody minded – he was always quick tempered, even when he was well, but there was a hint towards the end of a personality change, and he was just being horrible to me. I'd made him some soup and he was very rude about it. I said to him, "Excuse me, I'm not going to sit here and listen to this!," and I stormed out of the ward! I came home and sat down and thought, "What am I doing?" It was awful. I still feel terrible about that, and that guilt will always stay with me, even though it only happened once.

My mother at that stage didn't know that he had AIDS, although she knew he'd been ill. But then in November I had to go into hospital to have major surgery, and Mark actually told my mother and my sister then. My sister was completely stunned to begin with, but they were both great. Neither of them wanted to know how he'd got it. My mother told only the immediate family – there was a feeling that we'd only tell those who needed to know. She was wonderful – she just told me to tell her if I needed her. My friends were very much aware what was going on, and my close friends at work, so there was lots of support there.

Mark had made a will – we did it together, as soon as we knew what was happening. We were really tying up all the loose ends. There were a couple of people he wanted to see before he died, so he did that too and that was good.

I had four weeks convalescence after my operation, and then I went back to work. It was at some stage after that, February or March, that he started losing his appetite, and then feeling sick. He'd have a good day one day and then a bad day, and he just generally got weaker. There was an awful lot of medication too – he was still on AZT and on septrin for the PCP, and the

101

recommended dose of that was about twice the normal amount, and he was on something for the toxo too. I can't actually remember all the pills he was on, but there was certainly a fair whack of them. The generally being unwell went on for a while, until we got to about Easter, which was when he really started deteriorating.

I think at that stage I really only thought about one day at a time – like any carer, I suppose. I'd cook him nice things, give him a smaller portion, eat less myself, see if he fancied anything, but I suppose at the back of my mind, looking back, there was always the wondering "when".

He got very thin and his eyes got very bulgy. We were both conscious of the change in his body. It got to the stage that I was afraid to touch him, or give him a hug, in case he broke. My girlfriends would come round after work, and they'd always make a point of hugging him, very carefully. By this stage he was painfully thin, really emaciated and haggard, and he could only walk in a slow shuffle.

And then about six weeks before he died he stopped all his pills. I think he didn't properly accept the illness until then. That was another worst moment. We talked it all through, and we agreed that it was pointless to go on trying to prolong his life. Without treatment, we'd try and make the best use of the remaining time. Coming off the medication was really his decision – he just felt the medication was really not doing him any good at that stage, and he felt he'd rather just take his chance.

We talked then about death and dying, and we planned his funeral together. That must have been in May because I remember there was a Bank Holiday. The neighbours gave us an old wheelchair they had, they brushed it down, and polished it all up for us. And I tried to persuade him to go out of the house, because he was very weak. He could potter around the house, or stay in bed, but I thought it would be a nice change to go out in the wheelchair. But of course he was totally against the wheelchair, he didn't want anybody to see him in a wheelchair because then it would be obvious that he was ill and he couldn't be independent, and all that sort of thing.

After he stopped the medication, he felt much better for a little

102

while. In fact it was amazing – I was going to work on the Bank Holiday, and he actually called me from the top of the stairs, and walked down to meet me. He was so much better and stronger that we then went for a little walk into the little park just round the corner. We sat there for half an hour, and then came back. That was a week or two after he'd stopped his medication and he hadn't been able to do that for ages.

After that there just seemed to be a general decline – he was very, very weak, and although we used a lot of the special high calorie food and drinks, the special stuff they give you, it didn't make any difference.

He was still coping reasonably well at home though, and I didn't feel I needed anyone to actually nurse him while I was at work. He could just about manage to potter around, although he couldn't really manage to do a meal – I'd leave him things ready. We had the microwave at that stage, and he was using that a bit. He was still able to move around, because I remember we went over to see a friend who had just had a baby. It must have been early June, about two weeks before he died. We went to the house by taxi, and stayed about an hour and a half, and got a taxi back.

He was up in bed most of the time, but there were times when he'd still be able to stand at the side of the bed, and we'd crack some jokes about dancing, and have a little dance round on a bit of the floor. And then that was it really. He began to complain of stomach pain, and woke up one night in the middle of the night with it. So I just rang work and said I wouldn't be in.

The doctor came, and Mark actually asked to go on to diamorphine, the painkiller. Nobody could actually say what the pain was, whether it was Kaposi's, or thrush, or whether the lining of the gullet was just being lifted off. All we knew was that he was sick, and he couldn't eat. I stopped work completely, and stayed at home with him.

It was absolutely fine coping with him at home – I think even if I hadn't been a trained nurse I could have managed. There was one problem about being a trained nurse though – there were times when Mark felt I was just being "the nurse", playing a role, and he was just being "the patient", and that I wasn't being the wife and he wasn't being the husband. But my argument was at the time, well, I don't normally love my patient and I happen to love you!

He died here at home. We'd decided against him going into hospital unless it became absolutely impossible for him to be nursed at home. Home was where he was happiest and that's what we both wanted. It was wonderful to be to be at home and not to be rushing to and from the hospital. I never felt he needed night nursing, although I used to be frightened of falling asleep and him dying beside me. And I was terrified of leaving him on his own, and I was very conscious when I was out that he was on his own, so I didn't get out very often. But the buddy system came into play then, and we had people down from the East London buddying service.

We had the Community Care team coming in every day, certainly the last two weeks of his life. They came through the Middlesex. There is a doctor and three or four nurses who just go out into the community. They get the commodes, the soft mattresses, the extra pillows you need. They're at the end of the phone any time of the day or night if you need them, and if there are any problems they're always there. They were absolutely great. They would come in, stay for an hour or so, sit and talk to Mark or to me, occasionally have some lunch or something, and help like that. They also obviously helped with the medication. They go along with whatever wishes and plans you have – certainly when Mark decided to go on to medication again to stop the pain, even though it might kill him in the end, they didn't try and stop him at all.

Before he got really ill they used to visit once a week, and then they'd assess the situation, and if they decided they didn't need to come for a month they'd leave it for you to ring them when you needed them. I think Mark could have stayed at home even without them, but I would have needed some back-up with the medication. In the end that was all I was giving him, just the medication.

On his last night my friend and I stayed up with him all night, and he got a bit distressed at five o'clock in the morning. He'd actually been incontinent, and that was when we thought something might be going on. I phoned the nurse who was on call and she came over. She got here at about six and by that time his breathing was quite difficult. She just gave him something to settle him down, and he was basically unconscious at that stage. So the end was very peaceful, no pain.

The formalities were very easy – I'd been put in touch with a funeral parlour that dealt with people with AIDS, which is a big concern because some of them won't. Or at least they didn't then, I'm sure most of them do now. So I'd been in touch a couple of days before, basically just to decide on what sort of coffin to have, how many cars, what the procedure would be.

Because it was a Friday, I had to get him registered more or less straightaway, because otherwise you're looking at Monday before you can register. He died at a quarter to twelve, and by two o'clock I was in my friend's car and down to Bow Road to have him registered. I'd phoned up the doctor, and he came to do the death certificate. I kept Mark in the house till about five o'clock, and the undertakers came when I felt I was ready to let him go. They were very, very kind, and reverent and respectful.

We had the funeral at Edmonton where we'd got married, and his best friend officiated. We had the full Mass – he was Anglican but I'm a Catholic. He was cremated – that's what he wanted – and we scattered his ashes at Edmonton as well.

I went to Ireland a week later, and generally went through the motions with my family. My mother felt that was important – we had a Mass in the house, and the neighbours came, that sort of thing. I realised being with them then that the bond I had with my mother and my sister had become incredibly strong. We'd really built up something extra, something we can all rely on. And my mother, who's a real Irish earth-mother type, is now involved in quilt-making for AIDS-related charities in Ireland, which is great.

I came back home for a couple of weeks and then went back to work. I wanted a longer time off, but what with holiday arrangements and things I couldn't have the time. I didn't really want to go back. The first day was a bit hard – there were some flowers waiting for me welcoming me back. I talked to a couple of people about it, and how things were, and then work sort of took over for a while. But after a while I found I couldn't really do it. At that stage I felt I was coping with other people's pain when I was at

105

work, when I felt I hadn't really coped with my own pain or come to terms with being on my own.

I'd find myself talking to women who were in exactly the same position as I'd been in, caring for someone terminally ill, and they were saying, I'll be able to do this and that and cope this and that way.

I'd be saying, well you'll need to keep some time for yourself. And by the end of the day I was absolutely racked by it.

So I gave my notice in and left at the end of three months. Basically I made a complete break for six months, although later I went back and filled in quite a lot. I went and stayed with Mark's sister in Australia and generally got myself back together.

I did go and have an HIV test – in fact I had one before I had surgery. I felt I owed that to the doctors looking after me to be completely in the clear. That one was negative, and I had another one last year, and that was fine too. So there's every indication that I'm not, but at the same time, who knows. Occasionally I think about it – most of the time I don't, but sometimes I do wonder if I am. But I made a decision not to have any more tests for the time being – I don't know whether I am HIV positive, I don't know whether I will be in the future, but that's a decision I made.

I'd had a hysterectomy before we were married, so I wouldn't ever have been able to have children, which in some respects I suppose was a good thing. It was something less to feel sad about, one complication less.

When I hear people talking about AIDS I do sometimes feel like stamping my foot down sometimes and saying, you know, it's not like that.

So I often find myself saying nothing, in case I sound a bit aggressive. It's a kind of protective coating, I suppose, I try not to give off an aura of knowing much more than anyone else about the illness. I do try and be objective when I'm talking to people, when people make statements like they still do. I hope that people are getting better educated about it and that things are changing and people becoming more understanding and less prejudiced.

Initially I felt I might like to get involved in working with AIDS patients, but all I felt at the end of it all was that I wanted to remove myself away from it altogether for as long as possible. You get to a stage when you feel your life is completely surrounded by it, it's part of your every conscious thought.

Now I'm doing a two-year nursing contract in Hong Kong which couldn't be much further away. It's been good sustenance for the soul.

PETER lived in London and worked as a clerical officer with the DSS. He was gay. His parents, RAY AND DEBORAH, were on the point of retirement when Peter was diagnosed as HIV positive. With incredible courage he allowed them to move house from London to Cumbria without telling them of his diagnosis. His parents went up to London whenever there was a crisis and he was in hospital, and were in London when he died at the age of 30. They are devout Catholics and have survived the ordeal partly because of their strong faith. Both of them took part in a feature I made for Woman's Hour *– as they live in Carlisle, we had to record it down the line from the local radio station, which was a courageous thing to do. A large part of their life now is given over to doing as much as they possibly can to help other people in similar situations, by going into schools, talking on local radio, and indeed contributing to this book.*

DEBORAH

Peter told us he was gay when he was sixteen, so we'd come to terms with that. We had retired to the North of England, and Peter, even though he knew he was ill, didn't tell us in case we changed our plans and stayed in London with him. Six weeks after we moved, he came to stay for the weekend to tell us he had AIDS, it was very very traumatic. It was hard to believe, and hard to understand. I didn't know anything about it, and I didn't *want* to know.

I suppose we were typical as a family – it couldn't happen to us.

107

But Peter talked us through it when he first told us. We talked about how we could cope. He was very good. And then he went back to London and left us to come to terms with it – because it's a thing that every individual has to come to terms with differently. He was very brave. He did everything he could to put us in the picture, and we felt fortunate in having him. He was the one who took the lead, he was the one who guided us.

I think Ray looked at it differently in the beginning – I feel that the mother's love for a son is more of a love instinct. Peter and I were very close, and we talked about everything. I think I found it easier to talk to him than Ray did, but once we fully understood exactly what the situation was, we were all three in it together. In fact we became much closer. We knew that what Peter wanted from us was love and support – to be his parents.

RAY

Every father wants his son to be a big macho fellow, so when Peter told us he had AIDS, it was like a bolt from the blue. I think he found it hard to tell us; I think he felt he was letting us down. He was very honest, and didn't want to hold anything back. That was a trait in him which went right through his life.

When he told us he had AIDS I was afraid – after all, he'd just broken the news that he was going to die. I was angry, but Peter knew I would be angry at first, and accepted it. I wasn't angry with Peter, but I was angry that he was going to die. He went home and left us to chew it over. And when it sank in, although I was still angry, I think I loved him more, as if I was given that love to compensate for what I was going to lose.

We guessed how he'd got it, he didn't need to explain it, and that was never a problem between us. We'd guessed what his life style was, so we'd half expected something to happen. And at the time he told us of the diagnosis, he wasn't ill. We wanted him to come and live with us, but he was sure that he was better off living in London where he could get the best support. And after we'd talked it through, we accepted that was true. We knew he had a wide circle of friends, and that London was the place where he could get the maximum amount of information.

The trouble was we just didn't know anything about AIDS, we were ignorant, and we just didn't realise all the implications. And there was no one up here we could go to for information – it really is a desert up here. We went to our family doctor, who said to me that he didn't know anything about it, and actually said that to him it was like leprosy!

Basically, we relied on Peter to give us information about the illness and what we could expect. He spent three days on the phone in the early days, trying to get us help locally, and eventually he came up with the lovely Adrienne, who was for a short time HIV co-ordinator for Carlisle. She came and saw us and sat and talked with us about AIDS. That helped a lot with our initial fears – we talked about what it was.

I feel that the literature the Government put out at the beginning of the epidemic was too scary – it made people needlessly frightened. We never thought about catching it – Peter just told us straight out that we couldn't. We coped in the beginning by walking, and talking to each other.

We visited him in London as often as we could, and really we got our support from Peter and from his friends. It's a terrible journey from Cumbria to London – five hours on the train, but it was worth it every time. And then Peter organised for us to go to a workshop organised by CARA, London Lighthouse, and Kensington and Chelsea Council. There were all sorts of people there – nurses, welfare people – we were the only two parents taking part which felt a bit odd. But we did find it helpful – people were so kind.

And we were all supported tremendously by the Sisters from the Convent of the Sacred Heart of Jesus in Carlisle. Peter met them at a workshop in London. They gave us all unconditional love and they visited Peter in hospital and at his flat. They were truly wonderful.

Peter lost his job quite early on. In fact soon after he was diagnosed HIV positive. Someone at the DSS found out about it and a group went to see the manager, and said to him either Peter goes or we go. The manager told Peter he'd have to leave, although he said if he had his way he would sack the other lot.

After that he worked for CARA on a voluntary basis, although

I think he did get paid a bit. But basically he was living on Sickness Benefit.

DEBORAH

We also had a problem in our own immediate family. Matthew, our other son, who is married with two children, visited Peter and he told him he was HIV positive. And from then on our daughter-in-law stayed away, although I think she did visit Peter once in hospital. She said she didn't want her children to know, because if their friends knew at the school they'd be rejected. It was their decision, we couldn't interfere, so even to this day our grandchildren don't know that Peter died of AIDS.

I found that terrible, because although Matthew was supportive, it was only part of him – the other part was protecting his family. The children are eleven and thirteen, and it does make life difficult because I still want to talk about Peter, and what we went through with him and we can't do that. We've got to be careful what we say when we're together.

Peter began to get ill quite soon after he'd told us the initial diagnosis. He got thrush in his mouth and his first serious illness was PCP, that was Christmas 1989. He went into hospital, into the Westminster, and we went down and stayed in his flat and visited him every day. We were frightened all the time – he was very ill. But he pulled through, and he kept pulling through. For a couple of months he was well, in fact he looked lovely. Then he got CMV of the lungs, and then he was in and out of hospital having blood transfusions because he was taking AZT which was causing anaemia.

Every time we got on the train to go home to Cumbria, we felt, help, something might happen, what will it be next time? Peter had PCP twice within a year, and from then on it was a gradual deterioration – there was always something; he had thrush and diarrhoea on and off, and he had Kaposi's towards the end.

I remember once after he'd been very ill with something, he rang up and he was feeling very low, very down, and he said to me, "Mum I wish it was just cancer." The most terrible thing about AIDS is that it's not just one or two illnesses.

110

One of the worst things were the terrible fits – we felt so blessed that we were with him for the first one. It was totally unexpected. We'd been shopping, and we were out in a restaurant for lunch. He was taking so many drugs by that time, and he'd been a bit funny ever since he got up in the morning. He began to feel very ill – I thought the problem was his legs, that his legs were getting weak. But he said to me, "No Mum, it's not my legs, it's my head." And as we were sitting there he suddenly looked from one to the other of us, with a terrible fear, and he stood up, grabbed a chair, and said, "Get me to hospital." Ray grabbed him – he was bleeding from his mouth, and shouted for someone to phone for an ambulance. A man from the restaurant got a chair and we sat him down, and looked inside his mouth, and he'd bitten his tongue, that was where the blood was coming from.

We took him to Charing Cross, and they were very good. They did a brain scan. The amazing thing was that after it was over, he simply said, "I'm pleased that's over." And when we were in the ambulance going home, he looked at Ray and said, "Dad, did you think that was it, the end?" And Ray said, yes, he had thought that. But I didn't think it was going to be the end. He had two more fits later on – during one of them he broke a tooth because he was on his own at the time. The whole illness was very nerve-racking, and very hurtful. But Peter always told us everything, what medication he was having, what was happening.

RAY

Peter did get fed up – he used to swear about being ill, especially when he had no energy and had to be wheeled about. He always said that when the quality of life disappeared for him he'd go. We were warned that there might be a personality change of some sort, mainly because of the combination of the drugs he was taking. And he did change – he was a normally placid person, but sometimes he was very quiet and placid and then suddenly he'd get very short tempered. He used to get very irate about silly things. We were sitting in his hospital room one day, talking, and suddenly he sat up, and shouted "Clear this f...... room, tidy this f...... room up!"

111

We took everything that was thrown at us – we cried all the time, and we cried with him, too, and he always said that was good.

DEBORAH

Peter died in the Thomas Macaulay ward at the Westminster Hospital in London. He eventually had septicaemia, his liver and kidneys packed up, he had two forms of TB, one in the blood and one in the bones, and he had Kaposi's. During his final illness he refused to take any more drugs. We couldn't get over how brave he was. On his final weekend he was very ill at home, and on Monday he went into hospital. He was so weak he couldn't get dressed on his own, and had to be carried downstairs. But he always hated the food in hospital so he insisted that he went to Marks & Spencer to do some food shopping first, even though he couldn't walk! When he got to hospital they said he wasn't that ill, he'd be all right. But I had a real premonition that he wasn't going to be all right this time. I knew it was bad, so I said to Ray, we're going down. By the time we got to the hospital, he was unconscious. I was so angry – I thought I'd missed being able to say goodbye.

But after a while he drifted back, and he did know we were there. His last words were, "Mum I'm going out soon – don't make a fuss." When I left on the Friday evening, I said, "I'm going, I'll see you tomorrow," and he didn't say anything, just pursed his lips for a kiss. I left at about 5.15 p.m. and he died at 7.50 p.m.

We went straight back to the hospital and spent a long time with him. He didn't die in pain – it was very peaceful, very quiet. He looked beautiful – the nurses made a fuss of him. When he died, they put a tulip on his pillow and a lily in his hand. But the hurtful thing was not to have been there when it happened.

Peter had organised his funeral, and we took him home with us to his flat and kept him there until the cremation. He wanted us to have a tea party with all his friends, so that's what we did.

Throughout his illness, one of the hardest things to bear was not being able to tell people. We needed to feel safe with people – we felt Peter was suffering enough and we didn't want him to have to cope with people shunning him. So we only told people we felt safe with, and we felt that especially with the neighbours it wasn't safe. That was lonely, you couldn't go to your neighbour and say, Peter's dying from AIDS. We did have, and still do have, some very bad reactions from people, but now we feel strong enough to say, that's their problem, not ours.

We do have one friend who we were quite close to. She never discussed it, and when we ring her she's quite normal, but now she never contacts us and we have the definite feeling she doesn't want us there. We were really good friends and so that's extra pain that you shouldn't really have to bear. I suppose they feel threatened, as if you might be carrying something and they're not willing to take that chance.

During Peter's illness we heard lots of people saying disgusting things about AIDS, like, we're not going to touch that in case we catch it, and when you listen to that it makes you draw back. We couldn't say then, well, our Peter's got AIDS. Although now I would, and I do say he died from AIDS-related illnesses. But at the time, we were shielding Peter, and to have to contend with that as well as coming to terms with the illness was hard.

I wish people would just be honest and talk to you, but they won't, they draw back, they just don't want to know. Even now when we go to church, since Peter died and we've never kept it a secret so people there do know, some people still can't accept it. They're lovely people, but when it comes to AIDS they clam up. A church congregation is no different from a group of people anywhere else.

RAY

One of the worst experiences we had was after Peter died. We were invited to someone's house for tea while we were on a religious retreat. It was a beautiful house and the lady of the house asked us why we were on the retreat. I told her about our son dying, and she asked what he died from.

Something in me said don't tell her, so I gave her the details of the AIDS-related illness. And then she said, "Thank goodness he wasn't one of that filthy AIDS mob." You can imagine our feelings, we just hurriedly made our excuses and left. And that really hurt.

Even my own sister-in-law said to us once, "I'm not sitting in that chair, how do I know who's been sitting in it, it could have been someone with AIDS."

We feel now that we're experts in the disease, and we've tried to get a support group going up here. A reporter wrote a piece about us in the local newspaper, but all we got was one scrawled note forwarded to us by the local Catholic priest.

We know there are families up here who have it, we know there are patients in Cumberland Infirmary, but they won't get in touch, because they're frightened.

DEBORAH

Our relationship, Ray's and mine, has become much stronger, because we were able to talk to each other about everything, all through Peter's illness we were able to discuss everything together. And when I look back over it, the relationship we had with Peter was wonderful, I wouldn't have missed it. And even though some of the things we went through with him were horrific, there's no other word for it, we had a beautiful bond between us because he was so open and honest, and in the middle of the sadness we found joy in that. He was such a wonderful son.

It saddens us terribly to think that some young people suffer all this without love, that just seems unbearable, the hurt must be indescribable.

RICHARD worked in London as a teacher of English as a foreign language. He lived in London and was close to his family, his father, mother and sister SUSAN. He was aged thirty-one when he was diagnosed HIV positive.

SUSAN

Richard decided to give up his job as a teacher two years after he was diagnosed HIV positive, not because he was ill but because he believed that he might not have long to live and he wanted to make the most of his life. It's odd but right from the beginning I believed he would die, even though some people have lived with HIV for very many years and have stayed perfectly healthy.

I was living with a boyfriend at the time of the diagnosis and Richard told my boyfriend that he was going to have the HIV test, but he didn't tell me. When he did tell me about the diagnosis it was on the phone and it was dreadful. We decided at the time not to tell my parents because we were convinced, quite wrongly as it turned out, that they wouldn't be able to handle this information.

They'd known Richard was gay for years, since he was about thirteen, and they had gone through the usual stages of hoping he'd grow out of it, but they had accepted it and always welcomed his gay friends home. The wider family didn't know – the aunts and uncles – it was always very hush hush.

Anyway, about a year later we told my father and he immediately said, "Don't tell your mother!" A year after that Richard couldn't stand it any longer. He was ready to tell her and so he did. She was very good but I think she was upset that we hadn't told her. She did say to me, "You've known for two years about this. I never guessed and I always worried this might happen but I thought it was all right because nobody said anything." And of course she hadn't asked. In fact, in the end, she was the toughest of us all. She got through it just by grit, I think.

None of us knew very much at all about HIV and AIDS. It was early days – after all, London Lighthouse wasn't even built. Richard went to Body Positive, who were still very new too, and through them he met Christopher Spence who started the Lighthouse. He then got very involved with the sort of early pioneers of the Lighthouse. He also gave up work because he was getting very involved in counselling and running workshops about AIDS issues. He met David Randall when David was in the throes of setting up CARA (Care and Resources for People Affected by AIDS–HIV). CARA was set up to bring awareness of AIDS issues into the churches, to build that bridge. Richard ran workshops and he had some private clients. In the family we always say it was as if he found his life's work in the last three years of his life.

He found his community, too. He'd had a real struggle with coming out as a gay man; he didn't do that till he was about twenty-six. Suddenly here was this issue, AIDS, which was bonding gay people. It was almost like finding religion – and at the time I used to think to myself that I didn't regret that he'd been diagnosed HIV positive (this was before the AIDS diagnosis came along) because, ironically, it brought him into his flowering.

He had great strengths of communication – and he had a very strong ethical integrity inside him, although he could often be quite insistent and fanatical with it. But there was a crusader feel to him, particularly in those last years when he was doing his life's work. In fact, I remember him saying to me once, "God, if I suddenly found that this HIV diagnosis was wrong, I don't know what I'd do."

So he did acknowledge that his identity was very much bound up with that, that he could stand up as an HIV positive man in front of some quite large audiences and win them over to an acceptance of it through his character. That was really what his work was about.

The AIDS diagnosis came in February 1989. It was Kaposi's which started on his forearm. He asked me round to his flat and he said, "I've got something to tell you," and he showed me this little spot. He'd already told my parents two days before. I asked him how he knew it was Kaposi's, and he said "I just know". He said it had been there for the last four months but he hadn't realised what it was till now, so I suppose there was a sort of cutting-out process going on. He hadn't been to the doctor but when he finally went the diagnosis was confirmed.

That year he started to get illnesses. He had PCP but it was always controlled with the Pentamidine inhaler. He also had severe irritis which was terribly painful and could have blinded him. He always had to wear dark glasses out of doors after that. Then he got ill with diarrhoea and sickness and underwent dramatic weight loss. He didn't go into hospital, although he regularly went to the Kobler Clinic.

In December 1989 my parents were looking after him at their house but they had booked a weekend away a long time before so he came to stay with me. During that weekend I honestly thought he was going to die. Looking back on it I was much too alarmist, but I was on my own and I'd never been in a situation with someone who was so weak, who was in bed, who couldn't keep his food down. It was terrifying. Richard told me later he'd been terrified too but he didn't show it at the time.

I remember that weekend so vividly, trying to feed Richard cornflakes or scrambled eggs. On the Sunday evening a friend of his came round with her mother. Her mother was learning to be an acupuncturist and she went upstairs and gave him an acupuncture session. Richard had a tremendous sense of humour – after a while I went upstairs, and he said "She's really got me pinned down here!" and he was lying there with all the needles in him. And that turned him round; he was able to eat after that. I think it changed his whole mood, but I also think it rebalanced something so that he was able to eat. That weekend was a real low point but his health stabilised, very slowly, after that.

He stayed with me for a couple of months after that, which was a completely new experience for me. I was living alone by then and I was working. I'd never had complete responsibility for anyone before but we managed quite well. We were always close, and we also had a fiery relationship, so it was close but quite sparky.

After Richard had been living with me for two months and he was getting better, I decided that I had to have my own space. I told him (and I knew this was going to be very difficult) that I needed to have some evenings or some time here on my own. Living alone is probably my preferred way of living and having him here all the time – having anyone here all the time – was quite difficult, particularly as he was much stronger. I told him I'd like him to go back to his flat for part of the week, and come to me for two or three nights a week. He was terribly upset. I think he saw it as a betrayal and I certainly felt I was betraying him. But although I felt bad about it I really didn't know how to handle it any more.

He was frightened of going back to the flat on his own, and I understood that. I wanted him to feel he could come here as a bolthole any time, but he was very much a black and white person and I think that was also exaggerated by his illness. So he moved out. He wouldn't stay at all and he wouldn't come on an occasional basis.

He told friends later, who've since told me, that he believed I needed to make the separation. Just as he was having to let go, so I had to also and I think he was right. The pain of the prospect of losing him was distorting me so that I was always acting out of fear and I couldn't deal with him in the normal way. It was the most indescribably painful period of my life, not simply because he was dying, funnily enough, but because of everything it was bringing up in me about my own insecurity.

Richard was able to fend for himself until the last six weeks of his life. He kept his flat on although it was in rather a state and he had a lot of work to do on it. We managed to persuade him to decorate his bedroom and to put flooring down in the kitchen, but he never had proper flooring in the hall. He didn't want the hassle of doing it himself and he was too tired to deal with strangers doing it. After he died we spent six months putting it to rights to sell it, and that was sad because I wish he could have seen it looking nice.

Richard never complained about his illness. He was incredibly resilient. He usually felt nauseous and I think he'd often go away and throw up and we'd never hear anything about it. He was often tired but he never complained or rued the fact that he'd got AIDS.

He had one particularly nasty experience. One of the jobs he did after he'd given up teaching was in the AIDS department at Westminster Hospital. His job involved looking up records and he came across the records of an old lover of his. It transpired that this man had been diagnosed HIV positive before Richard's relationship with him began. This man had already died by the time Richard found this out. We don't know whether this man had known, or whether he had deliberately and wilfully not told Richard, but that was a very big shock. There was certainly a possibility that he might have known he was HIV positive and still have put Richard at risk. Realising that was a bad moment. That was the only time I can remember him ruing his situation – it was just such a shock. We were all so glad the man had died because if he was alive now I don't know what I'd do.

Richard enjoyed his working life in the last few years – he had freedom and he was doing what he wanted to do. He got a lot of positive feedback; and he was very good at what he did. People thought he was wonderful and he thrived on that and he deserved to.

Then slowly in the last year, he developed a terrible cough to the point where he couldn't talk. I'd phone him up and he would say "I can't talk", cough cough cough. Nobody could do anything about it except give him heavy doses of drugs which would have knocked him unconscious. So that was his cross if you like. For someone whose whole life was about communicating it was very very sad. The Kaposi's never reached his face so it was never visible to anyone, which was good. The diagnosis of lung cancer came in July of his last year, 1990, and he had chemotherapy. He slowly got thinner and thinner, and weaker, and cough cough cough, all the time, even at night.

Richard was always very strong willed, and I think I was always a bit frightened of him during his illness, because he had very clear ideas about what he wanted to do. What I didn't realise at the time, although I do realise it now, is that as you lose control of your body you've got to keep control of something, that's the way you are going to survive. I was so terrified of losing him, and I didn't know how I was going to survive it, so sometimes I couldn't see what was happening because my own fear was taking me over.

I was working in Scotland from Monday to Friday in his last few months. My mother wanted to stay overnight with Richard when he was very sick, but he wouldn't let her. He'd say "I won't get a moment's rest because I'll be coughing and thinking that I'm keeping you awake." So right till the very last we were never allowed to stay at the flat, except once when he allowed her to stay at the flat. That was a few weeks before he died. Anything could have happened at night – so my mother sometimes came and stayed with me. He was very, very fixed about it. It was about being in control of his life.

My mother said to him one day, "I've just given the sitting-room a dust," and he got terribly cross. He said, "I've been looking after this flat for years, how dare you!" And of course, he was quite right. If she'd said, "Richard, can I dust the flat?" that might have been all right. But we were not allowed to treat him as an invalid. His flat was his space.

On another occasion we were nursing him over a week – I'd got a week off from work – and I brought in some food. My mother told him, "Susan's brought in some food" and he didn't like it: "Without telling me . . . into my fridge!" My mother said, "Well, actually dear, it is for me!" So there was all that boundaries stuff going on until the last minute.

I became very aware of how easy it is to infringe the natural rights of someone who is ill, although it used to irritate the hell out of me sometimes. Richard and I had a turbulent last year together. The sparky side of things between us was very painful for me and I think very painful for him. To be honest, I didn't know whether I was coming or going. By the end of 1990, he made the decision to go into the Lighthouse. As far as he was concerned, it was for a week's respite care and only on condition that he could have his own room because of the cough.

Before Richard went into Lighthouse we hadn't seen anyone else with AIDS so we didn't realise how far gone he was, which sounds ridiculous looking back on it. He could hardly move but somehow I thought he'd go home again and I took him seriously when he said respite. But as soon as he got in there, the nurses very gently said to my mother that he should stay at least two weeks and that there would always be a bed for Richard even if he decided to go back to his flat. In other words, the end is near.

It was very reassuring to know they would keep a room for him because it had become difficult looking after him without the gadgetry. For instance, if he wanted to go to the loo and couldn't get there they have these wonderful bottles, which we didn't have. We had nothing at all in the flat – no special mattresses, nothing. It's hard to credit looking back on it. I don't know why we didn't have them. I simply didn't ever go and ask anybody for them.

If I was going to go through this again, I'd have no hesitation in getting myself properly equipped instead of having to deal with buckets and God knows what! We just staggered through it day by day. Normally I'm quite a competent person but I just wasn't thinking straight. And he was so much in control that if I'd said to

120

him, "Look Richard, I'd like to go along to medical suppliers and get this, that, and the other," I might have got into trouble!

My parents and I were extremely cautious about suggesting anything at all to him because we believed that he knew what was available to people with AIDS and if he knew about it he could have chosen to get the things himself. Also, the control issue was the lifeline he was hanging on to and we were forced to respect it. That's very tough. It was like walking a tightrope.

It was tough on us but it did us a lot of good. I think it was a salutary lesson to us in how to be loving in a way that we wouldn't have chosen. In other words, we had to love him as he wanted to be loved and not as we wanted to love him. We could not get rid of all our pain in a rush of trying to help him, we actually had to sit with it. I don't think that was his intention – he just had to do things in his own way – but the result was that we couldn't lose our pain in a welter of fussing. I've never quite thought about it like this before but I think that is the truth. It is hard to understand someone else's own ground.

I feel that I would be able to deal with terminal illness in someone else a lot better now. I regret the fact that I had to learn it through my brother because I would have loved to have done better by him than I did. There were things where my own neediness was so over-riding that I didn't do as well as I could have done and I regret that.

But over the past two years I have had to accept that it was part of the learning process and I can't do anything about it. At the time I was convinced that I wasn't going to survive it. I don't mean I would have died myself but that I wasn't going to be able to handle it emotionally. I was a wreck for five years. From the moment he was diagnosed HIV positive I was in floods of tears all the time! I have survived, of course, and that knowledge alone would make me stronger next time. I know that I'm not going to be obliterated because of a tragedy like this.

I'd always played the role with Richard of being a resource for him to come to when he was in trouble. In that last year he refused to do that and it was hard for me to give up that role. He was basically saying to me "You've been my older, bossy sister all these years and I'm not going to let you do that any more!" and that was the lesson I had to learn. It was very difficult and it meant not seeing him for quite long periods of time in that last year because neither of us could handle it. He didn't want to see me because I couldn't hold the line of not doing the bossing, and I was terrified of seeing him because there was always the possibility of an explosion. It was only in the last few weeks that we had a really long talk about it.

I went round to see him and he said to me, "You have got to stop this", and I promised I would. And for the last few weeks it was different. There was one funny little incident. About five days before he died I was tidying up something in his room and I'd done it wrong. He commented on it and I tightened my lips – I was consciously trying not to explode! And he turned to me cool as a cucumber and said, "I'm still a challenge to you, aren't I?" and I looked at him and laughed and said, "Yes, you are!" It's a very hard lesson to learn but he was a teacher for me in that last year.

Although I was half aware of these things going on at the time it's only since he died that I've been able to think it through properly. I think it was very hard to understand exactly what he was going through in facing his own death, in giving up his hopes for the future. It was too painful for me to contemplate.

When he went into the Lighthouse, it was just before Christmas. He had everything just as he wanted it – it was wonderful really. He had his Christmas tree with red baubles and white lights. I scoured London for those red balls and white lights and I decorated the tree under his instructions! He had all his things just as he wanted them and I look back on that time very fondly. It was a stressful time trying to tiptoe round what he wanted, but it was good.

We had the Sunday before Christmas at CARA, which is just opposite Lighthouse. He was very ill but we wheeled him over in his dressing-gown and he sat there in the midst of his friends. We had a lovely meal and we sang carols. Afterwards when I was washing-up I knew that Richard was in the other room being looked after and loved, it was wonderful!

There are some very precious memories of that time. Because he was fading away he got more and more translucent. He was very thin but his illness didn't show on his face, but he looked more and more ascetic and – it's a funny word to use – holy really. There were some absolutely wonderful moments. I remember bringing him a bunch of jasmine from my garden and I'd arranged them and put them against the wall. The nurse came in and he said to her, "Do you like my flowers, they're from my sister's garden". It was so gentle and lovely and he really appreciated them. I hadn't realised how much he had enjoyed looking at them.

The Lighthouse nurses were wonderful. There were eight of them on Richard's "team", which confused him at first. It took him about four days to get comfortable with all the different faces. But then he settled in and became very attached indeed to two or three of them. As a family we have nothing but praise for them.

One thing troubled us though, because it upset Richard so much. The Lighthouse has a policy of keeping residents fully informed about their health and medication, which is basically good. However, in his last two weeks, Richard was terrified that the virus had got to his brain because he was beginning to forget things. He asked the doctor whether this might be the case and the doctor told him it was a possibility. Richard was very frightened by that. He thought he was going mad, and for the following week one of us stayed the night with him in his room because he was frightened of waking up and not knowing where he was or who was with him.

But the fact was Richard had just been put on a heavy cocktail of drugs and it wasn't surprising that he was getting forgetful. Richard though was convinced he might have dementia, which is one of the things people with AIDS fear most, and he was terrified. So, at the very least, the information was handled badly by the doctor and we were angry that Richard had to bear unnecessary fears in the last days of his life. Two years on I still feel there must be some better way of reconciling the policy of telling the truth with the dying person's emotional needs.

Richard made his will about two weeks before he died. He sorted out his funeral with a priest friend of his. It was all quite last minute. We had talked about his estate a bit and he said to me, "The only good thing about this is that I'll be able to leave Mum and Dad some money."

He died on the 4th January 1991. On New Year's Eve he and I spent the evening together. We had the television on and he was quite alert. We had a nice evening. We just sat there, rather like an old married couple passing the time of day. It was very, very nice – we'd sit, and then talk a bit. After New Year he went downhill very very quickly. It was almost as if he had to get past New Year.

The nurses always told him what they were going to do to him even when he was lying there asleep. My mother and I would say "Do they have to keep disturbing him like this?" They would come in and say loudly "RICHARD! Just going to give you some more morphine." I remember on this last day which was the 3rd January, the nurse bent over him and said "RICHARD – ARE YOU IN PAIN?" and Richard shouted back very loudly "NO!".

It was the first thing he'd actually said that day and I'd assumed he was unconscious! I laugh about that now – but at the time of course it was a great comfort because he was a bit restless and we couldn't be sure that he wasn't in pain. So clearly he was in that state of letting go into something else.

He was on morphine for twenty-four hours before he died. It was a very neat little thing, the morphine, a bit like a small Walkman, and the needle just slipped into the hip. You could squeeze it to give a boost of morphine. We never did, actually. I remember washing his mouth out on that last day with that special little thing they have and he finally got fed up with it and pushed it away. He knew what I was doing so I think he was sometimes there and sometimes not there. He definitely wasn't in a coma.

My mother and I were in the room when he died. About an hour before I'd wanted to know what would happen when he died because I'd heard all this stuff about body bags and I wanted to be prepared. I found a nurse and asked her what really happened. She told me there was nothing like that. She then said she thought I ought to go and get a good night's rest and offered to make a bed up for me in another room. "No," I said, "I must be in there with him."

She told me that he might go on for another two weeks, he was strong, he was young, he had a very strong heart. I said, "Tomorrow night you can make me up a bed, but tonight I'm going to be in there." I had taken in a folding bed from my home and I was lying down on that at the foot of the bed and my mother was sitting in the armchair beside the bed. My father was in the conservatory nearby, sleeping in an armchair.

I'd been asleep for ten minutes and Mum suddenly jumped up and said, "He's stopped breathing". I remember getting up and looking at him and saying, "No, he's all right". I lay down again and dropped off but she knew he had died. And it was very odd – the nurse came in without being called and she'd never ever come in before without being called. Afterwards we asked her why she came in then and she said, "I don't know, something just made me." She confirmed that he had died.

It was a very peaceful going. He just slipped away. He had been terrified of how he was going to die; he had confided to me that he had a big fear of choking to death. But in the end he got the peaceful death he had longed for.

Richard died at 1.20 a.m., and we sat with his body for a few hours. We came out of the Lighthouse at about eight o'clock in the morning. It was a beautiful day. It was cold, crisp and sunny and I remember feeling exactly as though I'd lost a leg or an arm. I felt like an amputee. I felt this for about eighteen months – as if the three of us had lost a limb and we'd always be crippled because of it. It's only in the last few months that I feel that the three of us, my parents and I, have reconfigured into a whole again. We'll never forget him and we talk about him all the time, but we are now a whole unit again. I don't know what my parents felt, but I felt we were always missing the leg we'd lost. It was like an emotional amputation.

The Lighthouse were brilliant with all the formalities and arrangements. But when my parents went to register the death, the Registrar began asking them all sorts of questions about Richard, how old he was, his occupation, and so on. Eventually, my father asked what these questions were for and the Registrar said they liked to keep their statistics up-to-date, although it wasn't a statutory obligation. I thought, dear God, here are two parents who have lost their son the day before. Talk about insensitivity! I was shocked, I thought that was terrible.

About two years before Richard died, when the AIDS diagnosis came through, my parents had told the wider family – the uncles and aunts and cousins – that he was gay and had AIDS, and they were very sympathetic and supportive. My mother is still selective about saying what he died of – she's got a series of things she says. Sometimes it's AIDS, sometimes AIDS-related cancer, which is easier, and sometimes she'll say lung cancer. I think AIDS-related cancer is the favourite because it says the truth but in a less bald way than simply AIDS! I think it's quite clever, it softens the impact. AIDS has got so much attached to it – sex, death, homosexuality, disfigurement, all the taboos stuck firmly around it, so there's an emotional charge to it which other illnesses don't have.

My mother did tell one close neighbour about it, but another of her neighbours came to the funeral without knowing Richard had died from AIDS and learned about it at the funeral. The funeral was very open about AIDS, about Richard's work in the field. This particular neighbour whom my mother hadn't told for fear of encountering prejudice was in tears at the back of the church when I came down to say hello to her. I imagine the funeral played a part in making her realise what it was all about.

I worked out later that I had about seven weeks off work during the whole thing. I only told my colleagues about Richard's illness a few weeks before he died. They were very understanding and told me to take whatever time off I needed. I went back to work about a fortnight after he died. I remember the Gulf War started the week after the funeral and I can remember thinking "Good", because my father was very interested in this war and I was glad there was something which he could focus on. I think I felt numb. I couldn't cry for a long time and it was as if I was living in a cocoon. I've had one or two bouts of depression in my life, when it was like living inside a veil. It wasn't quite the same as that but there was a similarity.

When I went back to work I felt dreadful. I didn't realise it at the time but I couldn't concentrate and I was very unproductive. I took much longer to do things than I would normally. I was thin, I'd lost ten pounds in the week after his death, I couldn't eat. Looking back I think under similar circumstances I would take more time off work. My colleagues didn't put any pressure on me although I'm sure they thought she's not much cop!

I was terribly sensitive. People could easily say the wrong things to me about Richard, things which were very well meant but which would strike me in the wrong way. I was very protective about him, no one was allowed to say anything against him. Last autumn we were having trouble selling his flat, and we decided to redecorate it. I was looking at some of the carpentry Richard had done and I turned to my mother and said, "He was a rotten carpenter, wasn't he?" Now I couldn't have said that just after he died and I realised that reality was coming through.

The three of us sorted out his things together – my parents did the clothes. I did say to them I couldn't face the clothes. My mother has a resilience in her, she and Richard were very close but she couldn't cry. I only saw her cry once in all that time. It was after he died and I was very glad to see it. But I think it's too deep for her to cry, there's sometimes a level to which these things can go. That expression you read in novels, too deep for tears. I think that applies to her. I think she still experiences the shock of realising that she'll never see him again, that terrible shock.

When I realised he was dead, it was a terrible shock – realising he was never going to move again. However much it's expected you cannot prepare for it – or rather, I couldn't prepare for it. Sometimes, in the months that followed, I would re-experience that shock but that hasn't happened for a long time. I remember once, only once, doing the classic thing of thinking, "I must tell Richard that". A friend of mine lives near Richard's flat and last summer I had to go and see her and I thought, "I'll just pop in and see Richard on the way".

My father says that Richard is in his mind every day. He says he thinks about all the good times. Sometimes he'll say something profoundly moving about the son he has lost. On the first anniversary of Richard's death he sat up till the hour of death, keeping vigil.

I had three car accidents that January. I'd never had car accidents before and these were all going at about ten miles an hour! I scraped one car, I knocked the wing mirror off another and I backed into something. Each time I had to go to our accountant who deals with the insurance and confess, "I'm terribly sorry, I've had another prang!" I'd been driving for twenty-five years without a bump! I was clearly very disorientated but at the time I thought I was functioning well.

I think I did a lot of grieving beforehand and people say that if you do that it's easier afterwards. I don't think that is true but I do think the quality of the grieving is different.

The nephew of my closest girlfriend was killed out in Kuwait during Richard's last illness – he was twenty and he wasn't in the army but had been trapped there and was killed in a car crash while trying to get out of the country. I went to his funeral and that was exactly the opposite kind of death, completely out of the blue, although he'd been in great danger. My father said, "We're always looking for other people's situations which will make ours seem not so bad, so it's very natural to be glad you had time to prepare, whereas this boy's mother might well have said she was glad it was sudden. She might have hated to have to anticipate it." I think the grieving is just as intense but when you're prepared the shock element is lower.

We do a lot at CARA still, we go up once a month. That was a lifeline, particularly in the first year. Very early on I was invited to join in and help to organise their monthly Sunday lunch and that was manna from heaven. Richard had been on the organising committee and I was invited to take his place. I'm very very grateful to CARA. I hope we've now put back in what we got out but in the early days I needed to be with people who understood exactly how I was feeling. If you'd asked me a year ago to talk like this, it would have been too painful. It's only in the last year I've managed to achieve some degree of detachment.

At first I wanted to plunge into being involved with AIDS issues but I knew I had very dodgy motives and I knew I needed to sort myself out before I could offer anything. I think it's very easy once you've been involved in something like this to go hell for leather into getting involved. At the end of the day, there is a limit to how much I want to go on re-living the experience, so I will always do some work in the field, but I doubt it'll ever be my main work.

My parents are the only parents who regularly go to CARA. They go to every monthly Sunday lunch. There's a gathering before hand, everyone squashing in like sardines, and there are introductions, a thought for the day, and a time for remembering anyone who's ill or who has died and then upstairs to eat a big lunch. It lasts from about 1 p.m. to 5 p.m. My parents give to CARA and receive from CARA. It's a community of people who knew Richard and who talk about him.

Fathers are often the ones who reject the situation and my father finds himself talking to people who have the virus about their relationship with their father. One guy's father came over from New Zealand and at his son's request Dad took this father out for a meal and they talked together about what it was like. My parents decided that they wanted to offer anything they could so they told their GP in case anyone needed help from people who'd been through it. They also rang up their local vicar who had visited Lighthouse and written it up in the parish magazine. They told him their son had died in case he came across anyone in the parish who would like help. The vicar came round to visit them to do his pastoral "bit", not realising that my parents had worked all that through long since. Apparently it was quite amusing to watch this vicar trying to find his role! But they did meet up with a group of parents in Guildford. They didn't need support in the way I did though.

I've come to the conclusion that my parents' resilience comes partly from the fact that they went through the war. They were bombed, they didn't lose anyone but they came very close to it and I believe that at some level they had looked their survival in the face already.

In the September following Richard's death CARA offered a bereavement group, their first one. I suddenly felt a need to work a few things through and there was a man at CARA who'd lost his partner, who felt as I did. So we asked CARA if a group could be set up and they found someone to run it.

It was once a week for eight weeks and all the other people there were partners, not relatives, and I was the only woman. We were all at different stages of our bereavement – one or two people had only just lost their partners and I came to the view that getting people at similar stages was rather important. I'd already worked through some of the early stages but with some of them it was so raw.

If the leader of the group had not been so skilled we would have been completely overcome by this new grief. We did various things. We talked about our experiences, we brought in photographs of the person who had died and shared them, we talked about the person, we talked about our feelings. There was always some residual guilt and I had a fair mound of it to get through which had made me feel very bad. It was quite a relief to talk it through and realise that I wasn't the only wicked person on the planet! And we had some laughs too about some of the things Richard and these other people had done. It was good being able to say not only how wonderful they were at times but also how awful they were at times as well. I would recommend a group but I couldn't say everyone should do it because you do have to gear yourself up to it and it's not easy.

CHARLES *was a theatre director and actor. His father had been dead for several years and he was the only child of his mother* MARIA. *After university he'd worked in the theatre in the United States and in provincial theatre in England. He died in 1989.*

MARIA

I'd suspected Charles was gay and had talked about it to my husband while he was alive. My husband was a very relaxed, amiable type and he just said, well if he finds someone he's happy with, that's fair enough. We'd noticed that although he had many women friends there was no girlfriend.

Charles and I finally had a show down about it when I went to stay with him in Los Angeles for Christmas and he presented me with Leon, who was his lover. He didn't actually explain this to me. I just had to accept this young man in a house where they were sharing a bedroom together and obviously that was his way of telling me.

He was terribly shocked that I should be so forthright as to ask him outright about being gay, but it did clear the air. After that he knew that I'd taken it on board and accepted it.

In January 1987 he came back from the States looking terribly ill and I must say I did wonder if it was AIDS, but nothing was said then. He became ill in the May or June of that year when he was working in Exeter. He was diagnosed as having Crohn's Disease which of course turned out to be wrong. He also had terrible genital warts at the time which caused him a lot of pain.

He took himself up to St Mary's Paddington and checked in there in early June. He was examined, and told that he had full-blown AIDS. I'm sure he must have suspected that he was HIV positive before that but he never said anything to me. He phoned me as he was coming round from the anaesthetic after having had a bronchoscopy. He said he was ill and would I come up and see him, which of course I did. It was then he told me that he had AIDS, which I had already guessed.

He was very ill. He was hooked up to a drip and he was very emotional and weepy, and we just cried together. I hugged him. I remember that he screamed then because I pressed the drip, which hurt! He was very open with me – he just said I want you to know everything.

The worst part of that for me was being on my own and having to come up from Chichester to London, and having the dreadful train journey back. And having come back there was no one to tell, no one to talk to. That was one of the worst moments, seeing him so ill and being hit over the head with the diagnosis.

I have to say that the hospital were very good after Charles told me. I did see the doctors and they did talk to me and explain the diagnosis. He had PCP at that stage and they did say to me that they couldn't say how long he'd got to live. I felt I'd been treated very well at the hospital.

I went up to the hospital every two or three days. There was another complication which was that he'd smuggled two dogs back from the United States. He was absolutely devoted to them and this created a tremendous barrier between us. I'm an asthmatic and I can't have a dog in the house, which meant I could never have him to stay. The dogs were his life – he transferred all his love and devotion to the dogs, they were his family.

131

He came out of hospital and came down here for a while and we put the dogs in kennels. Then I found him accommodation where he could live with his two dogs, but it was totally unsatisfactory for him. He stayed with friends then he moved on to stay with other friends. He'd never had a place of his own because as a theatre director he moved around working in provincial theatres, places like Colchester, Salisbury, and Exeter, but by the end of 1987 he was really unable to work. He'd had pneumonia, he was on AZT, which made him feel ghastly and he was really quite ill.

From then on his life was that of a Gypsy, really, finding places to live, getting Social Security, which was difficult because he kept moving around. I supported him financially when he needed it but I couldn't find him a proper place to live if he still had the dogs. His ideal, having lived a lot in London and in Los Angeles, was to find a little cottage in the country with roses round the door, close to me in Sussex. And he did manage it for a few months in 1988, he found a cottage outside Chichester. He didn't have a partner after he came back from Los Angeles, but he did have the most tremendous amount of support from all his friends, they were wonderful.

In the early stages, when he first came out of hospital and the dogs went to be boarded and he came to stay here, I was worried about infection. I thought, well is it all right to use the same cups and glasses? Then I read the literature – I had a very good book from the Terrence Higgins Trust, which Charles got for me. I thought it was important for me to learn as much as I could – I read as much as I could, I had to learn about food and nourishment.

That was another great bone of contention – the food. He said flatly "I can't eat chicken", so that was out. Then we had this special food supplement which we had to buy privately, which at the time was thought to be good. The food business was a total fad but you just had to go along with it. He was absolutely neurotic about food – at one stage when he was in and out of hospital, he said, "I've got to have three square meals a day, and this is what I've got to have, porridge and bacon and eggs, and then for lunch I've got to have a three course meal." And he questioned every-thing I did. I learnt very quickly never to touch chicken or raw eggs. On the one hand I thought that's something I can do, cook for him, but on the other hand it's extremely disruptive of your own life.

His personality did change; I think he became totally selfish. I think that once you become someone with AIDS, one of the philosophies you're given is that it's important to take care of yourself, to think only of what you do and not to consider anyone else's feelings. I think that's particularly hard on families and specially if you're the mother. Because however much you're criticised, or ignored, you're going to take it simply because you're his mother after all. You may lose your temper occasionally, which I admit I did do a couple of times.

Once he was staying with me for the weekend and he decided to go back to London with some furniture and some china he'd bought, and some bottles of water. He had to have Volvic water and it was cheaper in Chichester so he took back six bottles. So there was this man, who could scarcely walk to the end of the road, insisting on going back to London on his own, with no one to meet him at the other end, with all this stuff to carry. So in the end I cracked and told him I thought he was being bloody stupid!

I think it is very hard to be someone who is always supportive – it doesn't matter if occasionally you're not that wonderful supportive being. You've got to retain the strength to be able to cope, especially if you're on your own like I was, and there are times when you have to say no, I don't think that's a good idea, I can't do that – but then of course you suffer terrible guilt.

I don't know how or when he caught it. His friends have said that of all people they wouldn't have expected Charles to catch it because it seems he wasn't very promiscuous. I just thought well, he's one of the unlucky ones.

In the early stages he really wanted to talk to me about it, he wanted me to know all the medical terms (most of which I couldn't remember, making him think, stupid woman, why can't she remember these things!). After he'd been so terribly ill in hospital with the PCP he contacted a lot of people that he hadn't told before about the illness – it was building bridges. And so then he didn't need me to talk to so much.

I must pay tribute to St Mary's: they were wonderful – they really looked after him well. He went on to AZT after the first PCP

133

which made him feel ghastly. But at some time in 1988 he felt well enough to go back to the United States – he had a lot of friends there, and actually wanted to become an American citizen. So he went back for a while and got involved in various projects.

When he came back he was in and out of hospital for blood transfusions and then Kaposi's Sarcoma showed up on his face. That was a most difficult experience for someone who was outstandingly goodlooking and charming – he knew he looked ghastly. He had that gaunt haggard look of someone who has cancer.

Soon after he came back from America he arranged for the dogs to be looked after because he knew he had to get himself a place to live. He found a flat in Dolphin Square in London, which made life much easier for him. It meant he could see more people.

In December 1988 he had a crisis and was in St Mary's for three weeks. He had very bad candida and they thought he was going to die. He couldn't swallow, he was on antibiotics and morphia and I remember thinking he wasn't going to survive. That was the first time I was allowed to meet Michael, who was very important to him. He was (terrible expression) his buddy. They'd met through the theatre and got on very well together. I met Michael in the hospital and he was a lifesaver to me because he was someone I could ring up and talk to about Charles and how difficult he was, and Michael would say, "You're telling me! rude and abrupt, do this, do that". But the lesson you learn is if this is what he wants you must allow him to have it, however irritating and stupid it seems.

I wasn't allowed to help Charles to settle into the flat, it was his friends who went round and helped him to decorate. He had no money so he wrote to Habitat and ICI and told them he was dying from AIDS and would they send him paint and wallpaper and they did. The Terrence Higgins Trust gave him a lot of help with things like fridges – and although I offered to help him financially, he said no. He went off to John Lewis and bought a carpet – and said to me, "Well Mother, don't worry about it because I may die before I've paid the bill, that'll be it". He had a wonderfully black sense of humour about it all. Michael and his friends went round all the second-hand shops and at last he felt he had a place of his own. Michael used to shop for him, collect his Social Security, and take him to the hospital. Some of his friends were terribly theatrical and would ring and say, "Darling, how marvellous. I've got some strawberries, I'll come round and we'll have tea, and won't that be wonderful." Whereas what he really needed was someone to come round and do the washing up, clean the bathroom and make his bed.

He needed to be close to St Mary's for transfusions and for the clinics, there was no point in him living in Chichester. At the time no one in Chichester had AIDS. When I thought he might come and live here I rang up the immune unit at the hospital and spoke to the doctor to find out about all the services and what could be done, but it was all new to them. I'm now on a committee for HIV services and I know there have only been three or four cases of people with AIDS in Chichester. So London was the best place for him to be. I found that very hard because I wanted to look after him. I feel very guilty about that now but I did accept it.

I had great trouble trying to find a dentist here who would treat him because he had AIDS. The GP here in Chichester told Charles that he knew very little about AIDS. It seemed that Charles knew far more than the doctor. I phoned the genito urinary doctor to ask him what I should do if my son came down to stay for a while – and he said himself he would be glad of anything Charles could tell him! I talked to my GP after Charles had died and he said that everyone in the practice was hoping at some stage to go on a course to learn more about AIDS. I did discover that people simply don't know about AIDS. The ignorance is still appalling. It's because of fear – people are embarrassed, like with bereavement, when someone dies, people are embarrassed.

There were opportunities when I longed to ask questions and talk to my son, but sons don't talk to their mothers about sex, and I had to accept that it was not possible to do that. The relationship gets in the way, so all you can do is show by your attitude that you accept everything. And although it's sad for me not to have resolved those things, I know a bit about bereavement and I know it's something I'll never be able to do and I have to learn to live with it.

I had one friend I could talk to – but the reason I didn't tell

135

people was that they found it difficult to cope with. I was quite happy to tell anyone. I wasn't ashamed or worried about it, but it was the dismay of other people and their inability to cope with the news that stopped me doing it. It was hard, but I could talk to Michael and there were two women friends of Charles' who were wonderful and took him meals into hospital. I talked to them.

Our relationship had always been a difficult one because we lived abroad when he was little and he went to boarding school, and we'd only see him for brief periods of time. So although I thought we had a close relationship it was never a question of coming home for the weekend and bringing friends. It would have been easier between us if there had been no dogs and he could have come and stayed with me. It's the times when you're just sitting around, getting up late, dishing up the dinner or pottering around the house when your children will say things to you and impart some piece of information which is vital.

I don't know where I got the strength from – I'm not a religious person but I'm a very strong person. I'd survived my husband's sudden death from a heart attack and two years later my brother committed suicide after his wife had died from cancer. I have to have periods of being quiet and just thinking things through. And I find that very interesting – a lot of people need to go to church, or join some support group. I tried the support group but I found that I ended up just listening to all the other people. When Charles was still alive I went to a branch of Terrence Higgins in Southsea; and there was a mixture of people, carers, people with HIV and AIDS, and I don't think that works. I could talk to a person one to one, but there are a lot of people who come along to these sort of groups as carers for the wrong sort of reason.

I'm in a curious position too – I'm a widow and I live in Chichester on my own. No one in the town ever knew my husband because I came here after he died and made a completely new life here and no one really knew Charles either. But I could talk to his friends, particularly after he died, and they were wonderful. It's three years ago now but they still ring me up sometimes, at Christmas, and say hello.

For anyone in this position it's important to have a good friend to talk to – the members of your own family may not necessarily be the best because they're all trying to cope with it themselves, but everyone must talk to someone.

The most difficult thing about someone dying of AIDS is that you have to put their wishes first, though you may not always succeed mind you! Charles did say to me on more than one occasion, "You're not being supportive enough." I'd ask him what he meant and he'd say "You're criticising me again." That had never mattered before, it had always been part of our relationship.

I found it very difficult that I wasn't allowed to be as supportive to him as his friends were. Obviously I rang his friends if he was staying there, or if I didn't know where he was. That made him very angry – and I realise now that his life was very compartmentalised. A lot of his friends didn't know one another and I had to respect his privacy and his control, which is one of the most difficult things to do when someone is ill. You want to support them, do things for them, and you have to keep stopping yourself.

Shortly after Michael had become his friend, I remember ringing Charles up because I hadn't heard from him for a while and there was this strange voice on the answer machine, "Charles is in hospital", and that was very hurtful. I thought who is this person? I hadn't a clue who he was – but Charles was ill, he'd had to go into hospital and he'd just asked Michael to change the message. You have to come to terms with the fact that although you're his mother, and he was the most important thing to me, I was not the most important thing to him. Why should I be?

AIDS is not necessarily a unifying thing either – you may be with other AIDS patients but that doesn't automatically give you an affinity with them and you won't always have things in common. I remember Charles being appalled at the other people smoking in the day room, two of them were waiters and there was no way he could relate to them.

One thing I learnt to be really careful about was punctuality. When I visited him in hospital or in the Lighthouse when he was ill, I had to arrive at the exact time – once I arrived one hour early and had to wait outside. Again I once made the mistake of going in early, and he shouted at me to go away. He wasn't prepared – he liked to be bathed and to be in clean pyjamas. He was an actor director, remember. I knew two or three friends of his that he

137

refused to see because they just turned up at the hospital.

Hospitals, particularly AIDS wards, are very slack about visiting hours. You can go up there any time and see someone on a morphine drip, or when they've just had diarrhoea or they've just been sick, when they're sweating and ill and they don't want that. I do feel strongly that hospitals should be far more in control of who goes in and when. I remember once sitting in the day room waiting because I was early and Charles walked straight past me into the kitchen and made a cup of coffee. But I knew better than to appear until the appointed time. It was the time which was important to him.

Death was never mentioned between us. It's difficult with someone so highly intelligent as Charles was – he must have known he was going to die, but at the same time he thought he was going to conquer it. That's what going to the States was all about. I think that after his return he'd accepted that he wasn't going to get better. But in any case by then he was fairly heavily doped so that he didn't know too much about it and that was probably a good thing.

I remember going to see him in the early days at St Mary's and he said the third time you come up in that lift is the last time. He did have this tremendous sense of humour – I can't say there were good moments exactly, but there was humour.

At the time though you're just getting on with life. If he had come down and lived with me I don't know how I would have coped. The practical side would have been fine – I could have found him a GP and the hospital would have been able to care for him. The trouble would have been that down here he would have been very isolated. In London there are so many other people and there is such a good support system.

We were both very aware of the possibility of dementia and blindness. You do think sometimes, because the personality is so different, it may be dementia. But by the last two or three weeks he'd almost gone into a world of his own.

I accepted that he was going to die and I think a lot of people can't do that. Although he never talked about death to me he talked about it to a priest who came here once when he was staying with me. It was someone he'd met who'd been a theatrical

138

designer and had taken Holy Orders. I gave them lunch and then he said, "Go away Mother, we don't want you here", and they discussed exactly what was to happen at his memorial service – he didn't want a funeral – and who was to have the invitations, what was to be said. That occupied a great deal of his time and it's not everyone who can do that.

The one thing Charles still wanted to do was to go back to the States. With AIDS patients you must allow them to do what they want to do. He was in the Lighthouse at the time, having some respite care, and he said, "This is what I'm going to do Mother, I'm going back to the States. Will you pay for the fare?" And I said "No, I won't, you're not fit to go, they'll never let you past immigration." By then he was about eight stone, I suppose, looking terrible, very thin, very debilitated, not able to eat very much. He asked various other friends, including Michael who also refused, and several others. But he got there. He simply used his bank card to pay for his air fare, and got an actress friend of his to take him to the airport. To this day I'll never know how he did it – he could barely walk. How he got on the plane and survived I don't know. By this time he was having to wear pads, he had constant diarrhoea and he had an ulcerated colon. I can't imagine either how he got past immigration. He did have an enormous amount of charm – a powerful weapon, charm. So he got there and stayed with some friends.

I was very against him going, not because I wanted to stop him doing what he wanted to do, but because I was afraid of him getting to immigration and being turned back, of getting ill on the way, of dying over there. But it was what he wanted, and he did it. He was there for a week. When he came back Michael met him at the airport and that was late July and he died on August 13th. So he'd done that so he could die. I realise now how important it was for him and perhaps I should have given him more support.

The last time he went into hospital, one of his friends who was visiting him had realised how ill he was and had taken him in. He was on a drip again and I wanted to rush up and see him straightaway, but Charles said there was no point while he was on the drip. That was the Monday and I planned to go in at the weekend.

I'd already arranged with Michael that he would be the one to be informed if something happened, since he was in London and then he could ring me. So when he rang me I went straight up to London and when I got there he'd just died. But Michael had been with him. He held his hand and was able just to be there while he died, for which I'm everlastingly grateful. They told me he'd had a slight spasm or stroke, I think it was quite peaceful, and no pain.

He had been in a lot of pain, because obviously he had cancer, the Kaposi's was all down his throat and in his stomach and goodness knows where else. They had at one stage talked about doing an internal examination and a colostomy, but they didn't, thank God, it would have been just one more thing.

But when he was in hospital he'd been on that wonderful morphia dosage where you have the little thing on your arm and you can just administer it yourself. He had it while he was at home and it worried me that – I rang up the hospital and asked them about it. But they give it to you in liquid form, a bottle of pink goo, so you can't really take an overdose because if you drank too much you'd be sick. Later I realised that he wouldn't have taken his own life – he was always going to go on and get better, that was his way of coping with AIDS.

Charles died on the Sunday morning and we waited about to see the Registrar, but because he wasn't the usual person he didn't sign the death certificate properly. It was like a sketch from out of *Monty Python*. Michael and I set off on Monday morning to go back to the hospital. We had to go to the department to collect the certificate and that took an hour. No one told us anything and then there was something wrong with the certificate again, so that was another three-hour wait. And then we had to belt along to the Registry office, which was quite Victorian. You sit in a waiting-room and you go in to see a very nice lady and the certificate has to be written out again in longhand. It's so archaic, it was a nightmare. But I'm told that was all quite usual, there are always delays. I was very upset at the time but I wasn't weeping and sobbing – it would have been a terrible experience for someone who was.

Michael took charge of everything after that. We'd already got the will sorted out, although in Charles' case he didn't have anything to leave – in fact he was in debt. But he had a lot of possessions, pictures and things. So he'd made a long list of them all, a whole exercise book in fact. I did say to him, "Look darling, you can't do this, you can't put all these details in your will – what you have to do is to trust either Michael or me, leave everything to us – and I suggest it's to Michael and not me," and he agreed. I think he wanted to spare me the labour.

This is where the Terrence Higgins is great – they send someone into the hospital to witness the will. The advice I would give is to keep it simple – leave everything to one person to dispose of as you wish. To die intestate makes such a lot of work so if people can bring themselves to do something about a will it does save a lot of bother later on.

The hospital dealt with the body. Because he didn't want to have a funeral I think he was cremated at the undertakers – the hospital have a list of undertakers who will deal with AIDS patients. Michael went and collected his ashes which we had at the memorial services. Charles wanted the ashes scattered at the place in Essex where the dogs had been found a home. I found that quite hurtful that he wanted the ashes to be with the dogs – I felt I might quite have liked to scatter them in the garden, but clearly they were like his children.

And that was another saga. When Michael opened the urn, to his horror the ashes were in a sealed plastic bag and this is quite tough when you're out in the open country – we didn't have anything to open this wretched bag with. I laugh about it now but that kind of thing can be very distressing on such a solemn occasion. So do check when you get the ashes that you've got some scissors to open the bag with.

I'd learnt enough from my previous bereavements not to rush out instantly and begin working with AIDS people. It was a pretty dreadful time. I spent a lot of time weeping and I kept myself to myself. When you train to work with Cruse, the widow's bereavement group, they sensibly won't take you on until two years have passed. Eventually I got involved with that which was good.

AIDS is still a gay disease. And the gay community is still not being targeted enough. I work for the Chichester Aids Network, we've been going about eighteen months, and we find it very difficult, although we've got two gay men on the committee, to know who they are. They don't always want to be known and AIDS is still more prevalent among the gay community although the numbers in the heterosexual community and among women are going up.

One of the men has told me that he's known three people in the last few years who've committed suicide because they were gay. The feeling against gay people is still so strong. I tend to accept it, it's accepted among writers and theatrical people – but if you're a solicitor or a priest it can be very difficult.

I'm far enough away from Charles' death now to work with people with AIDS – and I also think I'm pretty tough. I've met a lot of people in my bereavement work who are not able to grieve and it's very important that you're angry, that you weep and cry and talk about it to everybody. But finally you have to come to accept the fact that your son or whoever has died and you have to try and accept life without them. Some people can't do that, some people will always go on grieving.

Anger is a natural part of grieving – it's part of the stages of grief that Elizabeth Kubler Ross writes about. And there's also the cyclical thing – that you go through the anger and suddenly, a year later, you're angry again, and you think, what's happening? Little things will trigger it off, someone else's circumstances perhaps – here you are alone, your husband's dead, your only son has died from AIDS and you meet someone who's living a really promiscuous life, who doesn't care, and you think why has this happened to me? But that's the way life is and until you resolve the anger, you can't come to the acceptance.

KEITH trained as a classical musician. He had two sisters and his mother JESSICA was divorced and widowed. She comes from the United States and now lives in Sussex. Keith went to live in America with relatives when he was seventeen. He went to high school and college in America to study music and drama. He was diagnosed with AIDS in 1984 at the age of twenty-six.

JESSICA

Even at the age of three Keith had a great feeling for minorities. He always befriended them. I remember a Filipino road worker whom Keith called "my friend", and I remember it used to make this man blush. I remember also that when he realised that blacks were different, he wanted to be black. If he saw a cripple as a child he would imitate them, which was really rather embarrassing, but he was trying to enter in and wanted to know what it was like to be that person.

We tend to judge society by its sexuality and yet that's silly. The other night I watched a television programme about dancers in the Cook Islands – and as I was watching them I remembered how if you meet a man over there he will invite you to sleep with him and if you say no thank you very much it doesn't mean anything. He's not upset, or offended, it's rather like saying I hope you're feeling well today.

They are sexually so free that they're not measured by it, but here we are, we explain everything by sexuality.

I'd suspected Keith was gay. One of my pet theories is that not half the men who are gay really are gay, they're just not happy with the macho man image.

So Keith was trying homosexuality, I thought, going in on the side of the minority. I remember him saying to me a few months before he died that his gay friends thought he would survive and be married with children by the time he was thirty, in other words his friends also thought he could go back to being heterosexual. I think he wanted to be sexually active but didn't relish the idea of being sexually aggressive with a woman.

I read about AIDS, and I thought "ah . . ." to myself. One day he rang me from New York City and said he'd been diagnosed as having Kaposi's Sarcoma. I said to him, "Keith, why are you crying?" I hoped he wasn't afraid of death because that's not something my family goes in for and I hoped he had absorbed this by osmosis! He said, "Mum I'm not afraid of dying, I'm only afraid of the pain."

I found out later that he'd first of all phoned his father's second and by then divorced wife, whom he didn't even know, and told her! She quite rightly said, go on, phone your mum. I knew that was because he just wanted to put off telling me: he didn't want to hurt me. My first feeling was, well, it's just the next task. I'd brought up three children on my own, his father and I were divorced when Keith was about seven and that had not been easy.

He was then twenty-six. Keith knew about AIDS, after all in 1984 it was all over New York. I wanted him to come home immediately because I thought the doctors and their attitudes would be better over here. He said he would but he needed to finish his tests first.

He'd had hepatitis and I'd experienced that people with liver problems have difficulty making up their minds. My daughter had just started a job with the Greater London Council as a computer programmer, her first job; she sat on the edge of her desk and had conversations with him trying to persuade him to come over, but he couldn't make up his mind to return to England.

But one day she was talking to him about how the treatment was in such an experimental stage and on the same day his doctor in New York told him exactly the same thing; it was such early days. So that decided him; he rang my daughter and she leapt on a plane, packed him up in a day and brought him back here.

We then got him into a homeopathic clinic in Holland which agreed to take him, and they gave him treatment with injections of an extract of mistletoe. In the end they felt unable to give him blood transfusions so we had to bring him back through customs with all these needles for the injections, but luckily the customs people never stopped us!

The night after we came back from Holland, as I said goodnight to him I looked down and realised his fingernails were all blue, and I thought he might have pneumonia. So I knew I'd have to take him to my GP, and I also knew that pneumonia could be fatal, so

144

he might not be here in the morning. He of course was always absolutely certain he was going to make history and be the one to survive.

We went in to our GP first thing in the morning. He is a lovely man. He'd treated all the family over the years but he'd not met Keith for many years. He asked what the trouble was, and I said, "You're not going to like this!" Eventually I said, "It's AIDS", and he said instantly, "It's out of my field", but then he said, "How do you know?" and Keith pulled back his sleeve and showed him the KS, and the doctor put his fingers on it and touched it. I'll never forget that. This man is deeply religious, a wonderful family doctor, and he never flinched. After Keith died he confessed to me what I hadn't suspected, that he hated touching him. But from that moment on he never stood back. He said he would get him admitted to hospital as an emergency.

By some lucky fluke Keith was still registered as a National Health patient. Although we never took advantage of things like income supplement or invalidity benefit we did get hospital treatment.

Our doctor had trained at St Mary's Hospital Paddington, so he rang them up and they said we'd have to take him to a Harley Street consultant first, in order to be referred on to the hospital. We went up to London the next day to the Harley Street specialist. He examined Keith and seemed delighted to see KS, because it was quite rare in Britain in those days. He kept popping in and out saying he was arranging something with the hospital. I think he kept coming back into the room to look us over and try and assess our income. In the end he clearly worked out from our appearances (we were all dressed in old track suits and trainers!) that we were broke, which we were. Eventually he came back in and said he'd put him in as an NHS patient because the treatment Keith needed was going to be £3,000 a week!

We went straight from Harley Street into St Mary's. He was just getting pneumonia – and the hospital was used to that. The normal course in those days was for someone with AIDS to be admitted with PCP and die in a couple of days. I remember watching his temperature on his chart going up two inches off the chart. He had such a fever, it was quite spectacular. They kept thinking in hospital he was going to die, but each time he recovered.

He was in hospital about a week. At one stage they did a bronchoscopy and while they were doing that they punctured his lung! He was in such pain he fainted but they didn't realise what the problem was. The day it happened I was able to stay the night and I looked at him and thought "Well you're an interesting shade of purple!" When I went back the next morning he was very tired but pink again.

Apparently at one o'clock in the morning the doctors had realised what had happened and they all rushed in, put his arms above his head and a hollow needle into his side and let out all the air, and then that was fine.

I don't remember them giving him any drugs for the pneumonia but the doctors did say I could continue giving him the mistletoe if I changed it to an oral dose. But the fever he developed seemed to cure the pneumonia. And his Kaposi's all disappeared. I didn't know why that was but I wish I could have proved it was the mistletoe! After that they started treating him with Interferon gamma and then later the Kaposi's all came back, although I don't think those two things were necessarily linked.

It was an exhausting time, but it was also funny. I can remember the consultant saying to me loudly and very crossly, "I suppose you want to SPEAK to me!" I suppose it is usual at some stage in a serious illness to talk to the next of kin, but I couldn't think of what I was supposed to be asking him! As far as I was concerned we were struggling, they were struggling, we were shoulder to shoulder. It was the early days of AIDS and there were very few drugs. However, we went out in to the corridor and stared at one another like strange dogs. I didn't know what to ask and he didn't know what to say! I think he was expecting me to get angry. I'm a person who doesn't really get angry – I mean, sure, I get angry because the garage cheats me or a friend of mine. But I don't get angry about people or disease. He finally said to me, "This stuff you're giving him, you know I don't think it really does any good." And I said, "If the medical profession thought mistletoe could cure AIDS, you'd be using it!"

I do remember saying to him that I would never ask how long

Keith had to live, that seemed so unfair. Clearly the doctors couldn't know.

Keith came home when he came out of hospital. Then of course he had to start going to the outpatients' clinic in London twice a week. He had a wonderful young woman doctor, she was really good with him and with them all.

It was an exhausting time. The expense was horrendous. I never knew where the next penny was coming from, and I'd just started my job, where I help administer the accounts of four charities, a pension scheme and a private bank. So I had to keep coming in to the office to keep the thing going, because if you received a huge cheque you had to put it in the bank. In fact I did manage to do all the banking right up until the day he died, and then I did say I might stay away for a couple of days!

So Keith was living with us at home and trying all the alternative treatments he could think of. The Kaposi's got smaller but it spread further over his body. When people rang up to enquire how he was, I'd say, "He's reacting to the treatment." Keith however got the idea that he was much better than he was. He had some thrush of course and he was on the Interferon. There was no AZT in those days. But he was moderately well. He had a little job down here playing the piano for a little dancing school. Suddenly the two gay men on the staff discovered he had AIDS and went bananas, really bananas! That meant he had to withdraw from doing that.

That coincided with the end of the Interferon treatment and he decided to go back to New York. That was the worst moment of all for me. I thought I would never see him again. I thought he would drop dead in the gutter and I wouldn't even know he was dead, he would just disappear. I tried to dissuade him from going but he was absolutely determined to go. He said he had a lot of sheet music in New York, collections of 'thirties songs and things which he needed to sort out. I could cheerfully have set light to the whole bundle! Anyway, he wanted to go; he was determined to go. He was very stubborn which I suppose was why he was still alive.

It was spring, March, and I used to walk around and look at the daffodils, tulips and crocuses and think "He'll never see these again." At the same time I'd suddenly got a detached retina, which was operated on twice. It became infected and I had a huge swelling of the eyeball and nearly lost the eye. I did finally get referred to Moorfields in July, and the day I had my appointment was the day Keith rang me and said he was coming home. When I got to Moorfields they said they'd keep me in and do the operation the next day so I was out in time for his return.

When he arrived home his lymph system was affected and he was very swollen on one side of his body. Gradually it went through his system. I tentatively asked him about his symptoms and he didn't seem to have the terrible nausea which men can get when their testicles are swollen in Hodgkin's Disease.

We went right away to the outpatients' at St Mary's and he said, "Look, I know I refused any further treatment" (I hadn't realised that), "but now I am prepared to be operated on and have the fluid drained out." But the doctor said, "No, I'm afraid we can't do that, it's not possible." I said, "Well, it looks like we'll have to depend on the mistletoe!" And the doctor said, yes, that's right, depend on the mistletoe. She meant – think positive!

I think I was beyond being frightened by this stage. I knew I wanted him at home and I knew he probably wouldn't survive. I suppose I think it's immoral to despair; it's painful to hope, but it's more painful to despair. You just say, well maybe he'll be here tomorrow, and then you plan tomorrow.

Like Peter Pan, you know you're going to have to walk the plank and you're going to fall off the end, but you don't know where the end is. You're blindfolded, and you just keep walking. After all you can go out tomorrow and a bus could knock you down and devastate your family. We can make all the provisions we can think of, we have insurance, lawyers, we pretend we can know the future, but we can't know what is going to happen.

Keith knew a lot more about AIDS than we did. He'd read a lot of literature about it and even at the beginning it seemed logical that he wouldn't survive unless there was a miracle cure. That's another thing about walking the plank – the plank might be a bridge, there might be a miracle cure! We did talk about the various possibilities the illness might take, but it was silly to worry about what might happen. The thing was to watch him now and then handle it.

I think it's good for you to have to handle things day by day, to be busy doing everyday things like the washing; I think that's better than standing back and "being objective". That can be terrible. You shouldn't concentrate your energies on what might happen but on the suffering which is now and on alleviating the suffering, and enduring having to watch it in someone you love.

It's much better to be practical in life. Maybe that's why women survive better than men do, because women always have to do the washing. It's a whole planning process, you have to think: do we have the washing powder? how will I get the washing dry? It's like planning meals, men don't usually do that.

Sometimes when I put Keith on the train to go to London for his treatment I'd watch him totter off with his walking stick and wish for the train to crash. But, please, only that Keith should be killed and everyone else should survive. It would have been so much easier. Other times when I was out shopping I used to see young men of the same age walking about, and I'd think they had the secret, the secret of life, and Keith hadn't.

The next thing was that one day one of his eyes went; he suddenly went blind in one eye. So he rushed up to the hospital, complete with his juice machine and fifty tons of carrots so he could make his carrot juice. The hospital had just recently got the drug which could halt the eye condition so they were able to deal with that with a course of drugs. Then of course we were both one eyed; we had lots of jokes about putting things down on table edges that were three inches away.

He was losing weight because the thing about diarrhoea is that it just perpetuates itself. His godmother was a nurse and she told us to get this stuff from Boots, which was vegetable based and bulks up the bowel, and that helped the diarrhoea. He was still thin but he stopped losing weight. Then one day he came back from the hospital, and said, "Well, they think they can see a little spot on my lung and that's usually considered to be the beginning of the end, but it might be my nipple!" We didn't discuss it in detail, I said something like, "Yes, I see – well what shall we do today?"

The hospital said they'd like him in for three days. They planned to do a blood transfusion and then if his T-cells were high enough they'd begin some further treatment. I can't remember what it was going to be. I put him on the train on a Thursday. On the Sunday his sister went to collect him and she rang me up and said, "Mum he won't stay awake, I can't put him on the train. Can you come up by car and take him home?" I said, "With one eye! I really don't want to drive all the way to London and through the traffic with one eye, I don't feel safe!" At any rate, I did, and I managed all right. We put him in a wheelchair, and shovelled him into the car, where he promptly fell fast asleep.

I brought him home and put him in the chair in the living-room. He kept waking up and saying "It's lovely to be home", and then he'd go to sleep again. I put him to bed. Nobody had said anything to us about his condition, or warned us, which I found quite extraordinary. They had told Keith what was wrong with him, but he had been so drowsy he couldn't remember to tell us! In fact they had discovered he had Kaposi's Sarcoma in the brain lining.

For the rest of his life he could seem quite lucid but then sometimes he would hallucinate. But he was very forgetful. He would be all right for the first few hours in the morning, laughing like a drain, making great jokes, but we were used to him and we knew he wasn't being quite with it. Even in the good times he wasn't quite sequential, cause and effect didn't quite match up.

We didn't phone the hospital. I suppose we just got on with it and accepted that this was one further development. The next morning he woke up with a quite horrendous and blinding headache, so we rang the GP. He came and said that it was a headache caused by encephalitis and that it was often fatal in AIDS patients. I asked him what treatment he would advise. The GP said he would have to have diamorphine and I pointed out to him that I knew Keith hated to be drugged up.

So he left us with two things and said if one didn't make the headache better after two hours he'd have to have the diamorphine. The GP rang St Mary's who said, "Didn't you know? We don't expect to see him again now."

Again I thought this was a time when it would be better to be subjective for once, not objective. Seen objectively: here I am, a single mother, I've had this tough tough life, and here I am with

150

my only son about to die. I knew that wasn't going to help. I just said to myself, right, this is Keith and somehow or other he's going to last till tomorrow.

We gave him the dose of diamorphine, by mouth from a bottle. And then he just went ga-ga. First of all he went rigid with shock. He suddenly – in the middle of eating – stared straight in front of him and we were frightened he would choke on the food in his mouth. But I'd once worked with someone with brain cancer and I knew what the nurses did. So I went up to him and put a paper towel under his chin and I said very loudly "Keith, SPIT!" So then he chewed the food and swallowed it. And I said, typical Keith, stubborn to the last! He looked straight ahead and mumbled, "If you'd told me to swallow it I'd have spat!" (joke, joke!).

Then we had the breathing drama. He would only breathe once every twenty-five seconds, which is a long time. I'd gone back to work in the afternoon after the spitting drama and my daughter was with him. She was terrified he would die every time he didn't breathe. That went on into the night and then his godmother came. As soon as she came in he sat upright and said cheerfully, "Hallo Anne!" Then he went manic and he started telling all these dirty stories which he'd never done in front of us before! But she was good, she could handle it. He was just like a drunk, he wasn't Keith at all.

I went to bed and Anne stayed with him. She was marvellous. Apparently he suddenly fell asleep and then he went back into this peculiar breathing mode. Being a nurse she knew exactly what it was which was reassuring. His sister slept with him in the room, on cushions on the floor, and the next morning he was fine till about nine o'clock when he got the headache again.

We phoned the doctor and asked if we could give him some-thing less strong than the diamorphine, and he told us that first we'd have to wean him off it, even though we'd only given him one dose. This we did. From then on he was always fine first thing in the morning, and we'd have a good laugh together about the funny things he'd said the day before, like "Bring me that red thing off the windowsill!" His sister couldn't see anything even faintly resembling something red on the windowsill so eventually in desperation she mimed bringing him something. And then he got frightfully cross and said, "Don't be silly! Don't *pretend* to bring me something, there isn't anything there!"

One day he said, "I've drunk from the blue bottle!" meaning the bottle of diamorphine but we just didn't know whether he had. We kept it on the shelf and he could easily have reached it. Because he was so swollen on one side he fell over if he tried to get out of the bed, but given the position of the bottle I worked out that he could just about have managed to reach it, and he could indeed have drunk some. But there was no way he could have screwed the lid back on the bottle. The lid was firmly on, so we knew he hadn't had any. It was very odd. I don't think he was consciously teasing us or anything – it was more as if he was showing a kind of animal character, as if he had been slightly taken over by a more basic instinct.

He had no memory. One day I drove home and I could see him at the window, trying to get the window open. He was always asking where he was and when I went upstairs he was very excited. He said, "I was just trying to get the window open to tell you that I'm home, I'm home!" so I said, very over the top too, 'Oh good, that's wonderful!"

Another day he cut himself and I went to clean it up. But he said, "Don't do that Mum, it's dangerous for you!" I said it was fine, I hadn't got any cuts. It was curious – he couldn't remember that he had AIDS but he remembered the safety rules about blood from an AIDS patient.

By this time it was very difficult for him to walk. He just wasn't very interested in his legs so although we could get him to the loo and bring him back, there came a time when we needed to be able to lift him on and off a commode. I tried to get a commode from the Red Cross but they said they couldn't lend one for an AIDS patient. This was in 1984, probably before AIDS patients became top priorities in terms of benefits and things. I was shattered. After all, the Red Cross is part of the mythology of one's childhood, they're the people you turn to. Your neighbour can be frightened, the man who owns the launderette can be frightened, the doctor can even be frightened, I don't mind that, but for an organisation which means helpfulness, charity . . . how could they let you down? They have changed now, of course. I got angry with them;

I'm not quite over that yet. His godmother finally bullied a commode out of the Social Services.

Very soon afterwards he went into spasm. That is, he got cerebral irritation; the Kaposi's got a little too big and began to irritate the brain and he went into shock. His hands bent backwards, he went rigid. I rang up the GP and got one of the other partners. The other doctors simply didn't like the idea of Keith being at home being looked after by two women relatives! So this doctor was delighted to be able to tell me that he should now go to hospital. So there we were waiting for the ambulance and wondering who would come with it. I reckoned that if it was someone over fifty they wouldn't be in moon suits; if it was someone under forty they'd be. When they arrived they were both over fifty and they only had the smallest little gloves on, not even masks, they'd been through the war!

They took him into the local hospital and it became quite clear to me that the sister in charge of the isolation ward hated him, she just hated him. Not the nurses, just the sister. And I didn't warm to the doctor either whose name I luckily can't remember, although I remember we called him something rude and did it in front of the nurses too who never blinked an eyelid, so I guess they all disliked him too! I remember the doctor getting me in a corner and shouting at me really crossly, "Your son is DYING, do you accept that? You MUST accept it!" and me havering in front him and reluctantly saying, "Well, intellectually I do accept it but emotionally I don't, any more than the consultant in London would accept it." That shut him up.

By this time Keith was in a coma and they were giving him high doses of diamorphine "for the pain", but then he gradually came round and started talking again. Once my daughter was sitting with him, and I went in and she said, "Mum, he's been talking! and I've been giving him water." She'd been dripping water into him and sometimes he'd choke, sometimes it would go into his ear and sometimes he'd swallow it! We told him we were just going out for lunch and he mumbled "With the Chinese water torturer?" We laughed a lot about that and so did most of the nurses.

He was in hospital for about four weeks. He developed a fever and they treated it by stripping him off and blowing cold air on him. He hated being stripped off. The Kaposi's was quite extensive by then. I remember a gentleman from another part of the hospital asking whether he could take pictures of Keith. I thought I probably did mind but I was sure that Keith wouldn't, and after all he was still the one in charge.

The man asked him, "Mr Black, I'm going to take some pictures of you, do you mind?" And Keith put one hand on his hip and one under his cheek, the glamour pose, to indicate his pleasure to co-operate! It was so typical Keith – he couldn't speak, he could hardly move but could still tell a joke!

At this stage he had no memory of what he'd got, of how long he'd been ill or of what had happened yesterday. He'd say "Why am I here? am I having tests?" and I would say "Yes, don't worry, everything that can be done *is* being done." So he didn't suffer any discouragement. He was sure he was going to survive. We had worried about his having to come to terms with being defeated. At one point my eldest daughter became very fearful and said he was getting so weak that he'd have to come to terms with dying. I said we'd cross that bridge when we came to it, but we never came to it and that was very fortunate because it meant he was always cheerful. I imagine that he would have accepted it with grace, because he really wasn't afraid, but he was very stubborn.

The men from the Terrence Higgins Trust in Brighton came to visit him. They were delighted because it was the first time they had ever been to see someone twice! Normally they heard about someone, went to visit them and then they died.

No one, but no one, was in theory allowed to visit Keith but when the men from Terrence Higgins came they were allowed in! I couldn't believe it. Afterwards the sister said to one of them, "I'm so glad you were able to come, I don't like those three women being on their own with this boy, they need a man around!" At which point we really fell about laughing. What a ridiculous thing to say! And she hadn't even twigged that these two men were gay and, as it happened, HIV positive as well.

The sister really didn't want Keith in her ward. There was even one moment when she said to me, "Go on, take him home!" Which of course I would have been delighted to do; if I could have had twelve-hour care I would have taken him home with pleasure.

We did have the district nurse but he was already doing three people's jobs. He would come and do things like bath Keith but I needed someone for the nights. His waking consciousness was part sleep so his sleeping was partly awake. One never knew when he would try and get up at night. My daughters were both working so they couldn't stay up all night. I had tried to hire nursing help and failed – I couldn't find a single nurse willing to come and help me at home. I had rung all the agencies and they kept promising me they'd find someone, but they never did. I think they all just panicked.

Towards the end Keith wasn't moving so they were turning him regularly. He got pneumonia from being immobile, the sort that old ladies with broken hips get and it's usually fatal. He was only half conscious and I remember looking at him and thinking that on the whole it was better that he was not fully conscious as he wouldn't struggle to breathe. I thought I wouldn't want to watch him choke on it all.

My younger daughter by this time could not bear to visit him in hospital any more. She would have loved some counselling, but there was nothing of that sort in those days.

Then one day the pneumonia cleared up and that night he died. He was weak because he couldn't eat. But they didn't give him a drip, they gave him nothing, no sustenance at all. We'd left to go home because my elder daughter was exhausted, and I thought if I stayed she would too and she needed some rest. The hospital rang me at two o'clock in the morning, and said "Terribly sorry". I rang my younger daughter who said she didn't want to come in and see him. Poor love, half an hour later she changed her mind but her boyfriend's car was in the garage so she never made it. It was two in the morning after all.

We went to the hospital and they allowed us to sit with the body for about four hours, which was completely illegal because he was meant to go straight into a big plastic bag. One of the nurses had gone in to see him and she was with him when he died. She said he died so peacefully. She didn't like the idea of the bag but I looked at him and said, "Think of a chrysalis and a butterfly, there's no one living there any more. You cared for him, but he's not there any more."

155

We have certain meditations we do, like prayers, but slightly different because we belong to the anthroposophical movement, we believe in reincarnation and Christianity. We went out of the room eventually and they put him in the bag – he was so small and the bag was so big. They left him lying on the bed and they put a sheet over the bag and moulded it around the shape of his body. It was just like an Egyptian sarcophagus, very curious. Then they came with a trolley and put him on it, on the lower shelf.

We would have liked to have the body for three days before the cremation, but this was not to be. He had to go off to the hospital mortuary. I often wonder what it would be like if we had a society which was not afraid of death, which could talk about it. We have this absurd notion that we'll live for ever and we will not educate ourselves about death. We won't talk about it with young children, with teenagers. Perhaps if we weren't so frightened of it we might be more charitable.

We had the funeral and our own priest came. One of the things he said was, "Now the question we are left with is why should this particular ego choose AIDS as a way of leaving the earth in this incarnation." One of the men from the Terrence Higgins was there. He said it was the first funeral he'd been to where the cause of death was AIDS and had been openly mentioned. He was so pleased.

Such an extraordinary thing happened. The undertaker told the bearers to take their gloves off when they carried the coffin. Anne, the godmother, noticed and asked them afterwards why they'd done it and they said it was so as not to upset the family. I thought that was absolutely sweet of them.

One thing I discovered afterwards which I felt grim about was that the Infectious Diseases Officer at the hospital had arranged with the wonderful hospice in Crawley that they would take Keith if we wanted it. They were actually waiting for him, they'd even seen a training film about caring for AIDS patients. She had mentioned this to the sister but that woman had not mentioned it to us! And yet she had hated Keith. I would have loved him to be in the hospice, of course, particularly because he loved having people around him.

It's interesting to see that mothers tend to get a certain degree of strength after a son's death, but sisters don't if it's their brother. There's a fall-out among sisters: sisters do seem to take it very hard. Both mothers and sisters come to our support groups, but sometimes a mother comes and says "My daughter's just had a nervous breakdown for no apparent reason."

Looking back there's no doubt that the worst time for me was when Keith was in New York and I couldn't do anything. And of course as a mother you do wish you could have the illness *for* the child; it would be much easier if you were the one who was ill then you wouldn't have to watch the suffering. That was very painful.

The father of a patient in Brighton told me that the man in the next bed to his son in the ward had made the decision to tell his parents he had AIDS, and they travelled down to see him. After he told them they walked out and they didn't come back. That is the nightmare. It's dreadful – how can you live like that as parents and close your mind on your own past?

I still think that AIDS patients should be encouraged to tell their parents, whatever the circumstances, because the human being is flexible. Everyone is different. You can't predict what will happen. Prepare yourself for them walking out – that's the worst that can happen, there's nothing worse. None of this "I'm protecting them" – it's far worse for parents to learn afterwards.

My eldest daughter and Keith had a tremendous relationship during his illness, in fact she was his main carer, although they had quarrelled continuously from the time they were three and five. She'd loved him as a baby, in fact he was more her baby than mine I remember! But that stopped when she was five. Even when she was at university she really was having problems with her feelings of hatred towards him. I told her she was over twenty-one, she would just have to handle it. I really couldn't help her. And then a couple of years before he died, she went to visit him in New York, and although they drove each other mad by living in the same flat she did seem able to relate to him. When he came home and was ill she was everything a devoted sister could be, she did everything for him. She got cross with him sometimes too, which was not a bad thing.

When he had the intermittent breathing I remember her saying she wanted to shake him to make him breathe again! By the time he did die she was prepared for it I think.

My younger daughter did feel guilty about not being with him, although Keith himself would have understood why she felt unable to cope. He could cope with all sorts of sickness in animals, he was wonderful – just like a vet – but she never could with things like that and he knew that and understood it because she was his baby sister. He was protective towards her. Of course there was also a part of him that wanted the company, that wanted his hand held and his feet rubbed.

She felt guilty too about not going to see him once he was dead, and of course once the body was in the bag there was no possibility of that. She wanted to go and train as a volunteer at the Terrence Higgins and they said she could, but then they never got in touch with her.

In those days they took anyone, although now they wouldn't take her until a good length of time after the bereavement. So she could have gone and had a three-week course and that would have helped her a lot.

And that's another curious thing. I remember the first sister of an AIDS patient I met at the support group. She had small children of her own and she told me that just after her brother died she didn't want to cuddle her children. She didn't want to love them because she might lose them. She got over it, of course.

I remember when my first grand-daughter was born, I felt that same thing myself. I thought, "Thank you Liz for telling me about this – I know what this is!" Of course I picked the baby up immediately and cuddled her and I was fine, but it's a strange thing about this bereavement, you dread loving a small child. It is something to watch out for.

It was strange throughout the whole experience. I felt that there was no possibility for me in this situation to be a mother – I had to be like his brother. I had to stand shoulder to shoulder with him. He didn't want to be ill so I had to ignore him when he was ill, but yet look after him, but no cuddles.

It all had to be quite like the army, in a way. That was what he needed. Once he began to cry when he was alone with his godmother and when she asked him what was wrong, he said

"They're so brave!" and she said, "Don't you want them to be brave?" and he stopped crying and said, yes, yes he did. But he obviously couldn't break down with us. In a way you couldn't have Keith break down, he would have just collapsed completely and he needed to have control.

I often find myself in these support groups with people saying, "Get angry! cry! cry!", and after all I'm the American, I'm the one who's meant to let it all hang out, they're all British! And I end up being the one to say, "Look, self-control doesn't do you any harm! If you have started crying, all right, cry, but don't go round feeling you have to cry." A man came once and a very well-meaning lady suddenly broke through all the conversation and leant across to him, and said "CRY! CRY!", and he was appalled, absolutely shocked that she could have even mentioned the word! It didn't help him really.

On the other hand I think capital punishment should be brought back for people who say "Pull yourself together!" This is one thing that should never be said, and there should be a law against it.

I never wept while Keith was ill. I haven't wept. I weep for you and for those others who suffer but never for myself, and never for my son. If there is a God then I think it's pretty logical that he knows more than we do, and I do think there's a purpose and that life is not for enjoying but for learning. Sure, try and make it as pleasant as possible for everyone else but don't seek pleasure just for itself – ask what you can learn from it

Sometimes I feel a little bit sorry for myself, you know, what kind of life have you had – that's the old enemy, objectivity – then I think, come on, it's not over yet! I might still have tasks to do. After it was all over, I did get involved in setting up a support group. This thing had happened, it seemed to me the best thing to do was to spin straw into gold – take your nasty experiences and make them into something for someone else. So I go on attending the support group, and every month it's like walking into a cold shower! Sometimes I can help people and sometimes I can't, but I go along on the off-chance that I can help someone even a little bit.

CHRIS *was a haemophiliac and an only child. He was a distinguished model maker and military historian. Like many haemophiliacs, he needed regular transfusions of the blood-clotting substance Factor 8 to cope with the bleeds he experienced. In 1981 he was given blood imported from the United States and contaminated with the HIV virus. The blood was not screened. He died at the beginning of 1991.*

DIANA

We had been living together on and off since 1967. Chris was diagnosed as being HIV positive in 1983 and had probably been infected in 1981. The hospital keep all the blood samples and it was in 1981 that there was the batch of contaminated blood which was being given to haemophiliacs. But they didn't know for sure until 1983.

The diagnosis didn't have a terribly dramatic effect because nobody seemed to know much about it then and people didn't seem to take it very seriously. The hospital certainly didn't seem to take it very seriously. They gave Chris diet sheets but I don't think they thought people were going to start dying. They never told us to take precautions when making love for instance.

For four years he was absolutely fine. Then we split up, in about April 1986, and I began to look for somewhere else to live. We were both upset and we basically both stopped eating. I lost a ton of weight and of course it wasn't my business then to look after him. The hospital didn't check up on him either until they suddenly realised he'd lost about two stone in weight. By then he had pneumocystis and by the time he was admitted to hospital in about the November he was ill in a major way. It was really serious because he converted immediately to having AIDS.

Staying well is a lot to do with how your life is, whether you're on an even keel, whether you're happy, all sorts of things. There are other boys who are completely fine who are still HIV positive, maybe because they're in stable relationships and have very few worries.

He knew a huge amount about the illness. Chris had a group at the Royal Free for sufferers, wives and girlfriends if they wanted to go, and a lot of people got a great deal of help from that.

160

He got over the PCP but obviously it left its mark. He had to do the nebuilising bit after that, once a month if not more. He went on to AZT after the PCP, and then within three months he had meningitis really seriously. The hospital thought that would kill him, but it didn't. By then he was terribly fragile and very, very underweight. A couple of months later he had salmonella from which he never recovered properly. It left him with Slims Disease.

Then it began really to hit home because he could never put on weight, although he had all sorts of dietary supplements and things. He was always tired, although he bounced back a bit. He went on working – he used to drive himself to his studio about two miles from his flat – he had a bed there so he could get there and lie down for a while.

His parents were very upset and bewildered, not angry, not like I was. He got closer to them, specially to his mother. She would come up to London and look after him and cook him meals. He hated being alone, he really loathed it. So after a while I began to go round after work most nights and cook a meal and stay overnight. For the last two years of his life I was there with him. I was never really worried. I always thought he'd be all right. He wasn't that ill really until the very end so I didn't have to do any actual nursing.

I was there, cooking, and driving him around when he needed it – but he'd always needed that from time to time with the haemophilia anyway.

Chris had already had hepatitis three times, straight into the veins courtesy of the National Health Service, so AIDS was just the next thing that came along. Later on he did get terrible headaches when the disease began to affect the brain. The diarrhoea was awful, he was on Immodium for years, and then of course the muscles started to go. And all the time he was having bleeds, and having to go on having the Factor 8. At one stage I wanted to give up work to be there with him, but he wouldn't let me. He said he wasn't ill enough.

I never felt I needed support. Because I was so intent on looking after him it never wore me out or tired me. I had the office to come into which was great. Not many people knew exactly what was happening, although they knew he was ill. I didn't want to talk about it because I always thought it wouldn't be true if I didn't talk about it to people. Work was great because I had all my chums here and it was a totally different life. Because they were good friends I could also get quite a lot of time off if I needed it.

I didn't really want to talk to people about Chris's illness. It wasn't the stigma that was the problem, I just didn't want to confront it. People do behave very strangely – Chris always said that he felt that some of his friends abandoned him and melted away.

I never really read up about AIDS and although Chris would talk about it I never watched television programmes about it. I didn't want to know. I didn't want this huge cloud looming over me, dementia, blindness, cancer. I did know something about it obviously, but I thought if something happened I would cope with it when it came along and not before. That was my way of dealing with it – I didn't want to be prepared for something that might never happen.

He never developed dementia as such but the disease did begin to affect the brain. He became slightly irrational – he'd go out in the car and get very confused and not be able to find where he was going. He'd say he was OK. There was the time he went off to the Haemophilia Conference, which was in Bournemouth. He wouldn't let anyone drive him and he never got there. I went out to supper, came home and went to bed, and he arrived back at three in the morning having been driving since four in the afternoon. He'd failed to find the place. Even though he'd phoned them and got directions he'd still not been able to find them.

He'd managed to drive home to London, luckily. It happened again a few weeks later when he drove to a friends' house to play chess. He had great trouble finding their house and I had to go and collect him.

One evening we were due to meet some friends for supper but when I got home from work I discovered he'd dashed off in the car. That really did worry me. I kept ringing the friends' house and forty minutes later he still hadn't arrived – it's only a fifteen-minute trip. When he came back he said he'd been to their house and couldn't get a reply and by that time he was in a terrible state. The friends then came over and he was dozing off in a chair.

Suddenly he woke up and began talking about something we knew nothing about. Then he got really angry with us. The next day he was totally fine.

He did also have funny episodes with his eyes but that was because of the pills he was on, the muscle relaxants. Night sweats were very common but I don't know whether that was the AZT or the disease. He had tremendous problems with the cell count. They'd take him off the AZT and transfuse him which had a wonderful effect for a short time. He had thrush, not all the time, but he was on flucanozole for it so it wasn't too bad.

The real turning point came when we went to Scotland in September. He was very fragile but he was all right. He could walk about, very slowly, but he could do that. One day in St Andrews, he had a fall, a really bad one which led to a huge haemorrhage in the knee. That had to be treated and it made him immobile, he couldn't walk.

We came back to London and about six weeks later he got this terrific ear infection and had to go into hospital and be put on a drip. He wanted to go home for Christmas – he was absolutely determined to get out of hospital – he knew that it was going to be his last Christmas.

He and I never talked about death – he couldn't talk to me about it because I couldn't bear to discuss it. He knew that. But he knew that he could die at any time. He used to talk to one friend from work, he'd go to see this particular man once a week. He needed someone to talk to. He couldn't talk to his family and he couldn't talk to me. I was totally irrational. I would probably have burst into tears. It would have been no use talking to me and I regret that now. I was a wet dishrag, I could never bear to talk about it – I couldn't face up to it even when I knew he was dying. I kept pushing it away, thinking it's not going to happen. And then when he was in hospital and he was dying he couldn't talk. The disease had attacked his throat and he couldn't speak, and that was very difficult. Because he was on so many strong drugs I didn't know whether he could hear and understand what I was saying.

We got him out of hospital and took him to Sussex to spend Christmas with his parents – by then he was so weak he was in a wheelchair. The first day he was all right, he had a nice lunch.

163

The second day he couldn't swallow the medication, he kept bringing it up. So by Christmas Day he had lapsed into a near coma. The GP came and Chris rallied a bit. On Boxing Day he was hardly there. A friend came to see him and he knew who he was but he just kept slipping away. Then we got nurses in, a day nurse and a night nurse, and they were amazing. By then I'd spoken to the hospital and told them I couldn't get the medication down him. They told me not to worry, it wasn't going to make any difference.

The next day his parents had some neighbours round and Chris was amazing. He came round and he talked to everybody and sat up in the wheelchair, had some lunch and was absolutely in command. But then he had a relapse.

We called out the GP because his father and I thought that perhaps if we got him back into hospital they could put him on a drip again, it had worked so well before. We suddenly thought there was a chance. I really regret that now. They took him to the Macmillan unit at the local hospital where of course they're not into saving lives, they're just into easing you off. The minute I got there I regretted it – he kept saying why am I here, what am I doing here? The next day was New Year's Day, and I was in a panic. I wanted to get him home again but by then he was too ill to travel.

That was the thing that really upset me. He was in this ghastly hospital where he didn't want to be and he should have been at home. It's a huge thing that I regret. It was the wrong decision, but we made it because we thought there might be a chance to save his life. He would have had the same treatment at home actually because what they do is give you morphine and you disappear. He didn't seem to be in pain, but who knows? He was totally drugged – they put this pump of action morphine on him which releases something every half hour or so, so he wasn't conscious. He had a swelling in his throat and couldn't swallow. He couldn't get the saliva out and had to spit all the time.

He just got weaker and weaker and eventually he slipped away. I wanted to take him home as soon as it was over. By that time I was blaming the hospital for all sorts of things and I just wanted to get out of there. We got hold of the undertakers, a wonderful old-fashioned local firm, and we brought Chris home and he was laid out in the sitting-room. I'm sure the hospital told the undertakers what he died from and it was on the death certificate too. His father and I did everything. There was a lot to do – we chose the coffin, registered the death and organised the funeral, we were support for each other.

And right afterwards you're very very strong of course. His parents felt less strong but I felt that as I was younger this was something I could do to help them. Which was odd because really I was less prepared for his death than anyone else. I never thought that he would die. They of course had had forty years of thinking he could die at any moment because of the haemophilia, all their lives they'd lived with it. He'd been so ill all his life, he'd lost an eye and had a brain haemorrhage when he was a child. And yet all the time we'd been together he'd never really been dramatically ill with the haemophilia.

I feel bad that I didn't ever talk to him about dying and help in that way. But I couldn't, it was out of my control, I would have been no use. I suppose I should have tried harder but I also didn't want to accept it. I do regret that.

I don't think you do really prepare yourself for someone's death. It's pointless going round saying he could die at any moment. Yes, you think about it, but you have to look on the upside – most of the time he was reasonably well and you're not going to be a very cheery companion if you're thinking about death all the time.

You can't not be angry at the medical profession – how someone who was so bright and had so much to give could just be snuffed out like that – not just him but all his friends, when they were really young. That never stops making me feel furious and I can't imagine how it made Chris feel. Because he'd been so ill all his life anyway he'd had to cope with so much already. How do you come to terms with that?

He made a will the year before he died, the briefest thing you've ever seen, but at least it was done. After Chris died I stayed down in Sussex with his parents for several weeks and that helped me a lot because I didn't feel ready to go back to the office. I'd go in for a day and then go back to Sussex. It was Christmas, it was a horrible time of the year, bleak and cold. I had my friends who were very supportive. People are at first and then I had my work and then it got busy which was good. But I never wanted to go and talk to a bereavement counsellor – I can't imagine how it would have made it better. I've spent a lot of time in Sussex with his parents, which has been good.

I never worried that I might have caught the virus – I don't know why. I did go and get tested and I'm clear.

I thought the haemophiliacs should have got a huge amount of compensation and in the end they got a very small amount really. Those with families got more, that was only right, but considering those who were high earners I think they were treated appallingly.

MARTIN lived in London and worked for a wine merchant. He was diagnosed HIV eighteen months before he died aged forty-three. His father was dead, but his mother was still alive. His elder brother died from cancer some years earlier and he had another brother and a sister. He lived by himself in a flat but spent the last three months of his life with his sister SOPHIE in Oxfordshire, where she lived with her husband and two daughters.

SOPHIE

One day Martin rang me up, and said, "I've just been to the dentist and he suspects I might be HIV positive, because I've got a mouth infection which won't clear up." My father was a dental surgeon and we've always been very careful about our teeth. Martin's dentist is gay and he had other patients who had gone for the test.

So Martin went to St George's in Tooting, his local hospital, to have the HIV test. He went in a few days later, a Friday, to get the results and was told that he was positive, and goodbye and thank you. There was nobody on duty to give him counselling, no one to tell him what it was about, no one to give him a pamphlet, no one to make him a future appointment. There is an AIDS ward there now, and I don't think that would happen now, but I warn you, don't ever get your results on Friday! I think it was wicked of them.

So he came up to stay with us. We sat and we chatted about it

166

and then he went back to London. I wanted to find out more about AIDS, so I looked in the phone book and discovered OXAIDS, in Oxford. I rang them and I got an answerphone which said they weren't on duty till that evening – and I was cross because I wanted to get hold of some information immediately.

In the end the man on the line was helpful. But he couldn't tell me what the risks of infection were if Martin were to knock a wound open and bleed, or if he were sick in the bed and how long the virus would last and be alive in the body fluid. I wanted to know exactly where we all stood. I wanted to know that I could have him to stay safely in my home, and I could say to my friends, if he were to come to stay and needed to be looked after at the end, that he was living with us, that he has AIDS but you can't catch it. I wanted to be sure that if my daughter Lottie picked up Martin's toothbrush or if he left his razor on the side – she was only six, it's an age children do pick things up – that she couldn't catch the virus from them. I wanted to be sure it was all right if he kissed her. He was a very affectionate man and he was very affectionate with the children.

I was very open with people from the moment I knew he had HIV, I thought either they cut me off or they can get on with it. The news went round the village like wildfire, Sophie's brother's got AIDS! It's a tendency of mine in any case, I get quite a lot of satisfaction out of being blunt. If there had been prejudice, I think I'd have steam-rollered it a bit.

It was a bit difficult with my first husband, the father of my eldest daughter Katie. I told him that Martin had HIV and it looked as if it would blow into AIDS – and that knocked him for six. He told Katie that Uncle Martin was not to touch her any longer. Martin and Katie were very fond of each other – he was her godfather and we'd been up to London and stayed with him. She's a very intelligent down-to-earth girl and I said to her, "Look, if you feel you don't want Uncle Martin to kiss you, fine, you think about it, and we'll talk again." I didn't ever say to her, do this, don't do that. I wouldn't set myself up against her father either, he couldn't help the way he felt.

The best thing that happened for me was Princess Diana going in to the Lighthouse, kissing someone and holding their hands, because I was able to say to Katie's father, "If Princess Diana can do it, you have nothing to worry about." That really did help a lot.

The diagnosis was made in September 1990. For a while he carried on a normal life, but then he had to stop working because he just didn't have the strength to carry on. He was so very tired all the time. He followed what the hospital said to the letter – if they'd told him to stand on his head he would have done. And he helped them if they were doing some sort of trial, for drugs, or food. But after a while he began to feel too poorly to do that. He didn't go on to AZT immediately, not for about another six months and we never knew whether it was the side effects from the AZT or the disease that caused his legs to become very weak and his circulation bad.

He was sick a lot. If he drank tap water he'd be very ill twenty minutes later. It was something in the water, he'd always have to have bottled water. Sometimes he'd take the girls to McDonald's as a treat and if he had a milk shake that would make him ill because the milkshake powder is made up with water. He had to be terribly careful if he went into a pub that the lemonade wasn't made from a machine, that it came from a bottle.

He had thrush and he had herpes very badly, although it came and went and was very well controlled with flucanozole. But we got to the stage with the thrush that the drugs had no effect and it was very sore for him. He had nothing really major in terms of illnesses – he had one or two scares, lung things. Every month he had to breathe in Pentamidine through the nebuliser to prevent pneumonia.

He decided not to tell my mother that he had AIDS but that we would if she asked. She did in fact ask me soon after Christmas, and I said, "Yes Mum, he has got AIDS, but he just didn't want to tell you out of the blue." She and I discussed it and then he went to stay with her and talked about it. She had lost other children – there were six of us and there's only my brother John and I alive now. My eldest brother died two weeks before my twenty-first birthday, of cancer, and mother lost two baby daughters, one with a cot death and one was stillborn; and my little boy Duncan died from cancer so she'd lost her grandson which is almost like losing another child.

168

When you've had an awful lot of deaths you begin to think well, what's next? I think she was very glad my father was not alive to go through it. They had accepted the fact that Martin was gay and it had never bothered any of us.

Martin wasn't sure how he caught the HIV virus but ten years before he'd had trouble with glands in his neck and had gone into hospital and had a small piece of lymph gland removed. We were all paranoid about cancer, having lost my elder brother. It turned out to be nothing, but when he was diagnosed years later as being HIV his consultant said that it was a classic sign of being infected with HIV. So he'd done very well being healthy for ten years. He kept very fit, gave up smoking and he was very careful about what he ate. But he led a very promiscuous life, he was very honest about that.

His boyfriend lived in Switzerland, and he died the Easter after Martin was diagnosed. They were very fond of each other and he was devastated when Ernst died. It was a very strong relationship.

Martin really liked living on his own. Philip, my husband, and I discussed what we should do and Philip wrote to Martin and told him that he was welcome here any time. And that if Martin felt life was becoming too difficult living on his own in London we would like him to come and live with us.

We said we would arrange to keep his flat on so that he could still visit the flat whenever he wanted. We were planning to change our dining-room into his room so that he could bring the things he wanted from London. He could come and go as he pleased and we would arrange care here.

In London he had a home help who came every day. She didn't seem to mind what she did, shopping, washing, whatever. He also had two very very good buddies. One was an actress, and they enjoyed each other's company, she was wonderful. And then we had Sean, who was also HIV positive. His dentist Arthur and my brother John were also tremendously supportive. Arthur would do his shopping and come round and cook him lunch. And John would go round and cook his supper.

So Martin was able to stay in his own flat for a lot longer than if he'd had no support. He had terrible times at night, when he was poorly – he might have messed the bed, wet the bed, been sick in the bed. He couldn't even change the sheets on the bed, he was too weak to do that. That was the time he could ring up Sean and say, "Sean I'm in a terrible mess," and Sean would come round and sort it out. He couldn't have managed to survive on his own in London without that gang of people, and the HIV nurse went in a lot too. She was outstanding and she thought Martin was incredible because of his independence and his determination.

He went into hospital once I remember when he got terrible pains, just under his arm. It happened when he was here for the weekend and we were worried about it. I took him in to see my doctor. We'd just been to McDonalds and we didn't know then he'd be getting this reaction to the milk shakes. We hadn't been inside the surgery for more than a couple of minutes before he was sick everywhere, so she saw him in all his glory! The doctor thought he should go into the John Waring ward at the Churchill Hospital because they thought it might be a thrombosis. He went in for a couple of days and they wanted to give him a general anaesthetic and do a biopsy.

Martin said he'd rather go back to St George's in London and see what they said. He had great faith in St George's, because he'd been with them from the beginning. They tested him with a local, and they discovered he had boils coming up, in ghastly places, and they drew off all this foul stuff. So then they knew that it wasn't cancer, just boils and terrible pain.

He went in once because he had a lung infection and was on a drip. Every time he went into hospital he recovered, but came out a little bit weaker. I could see that. But as far as he was concerned, every illness was to be treated and dealt with and taken as it came.

He tried to keep very fit – he swam every day, right up until the week before he came to live with me. For the last nine months of his life he had no T-cells at all. When he had that blood test, he said to them, "Don't tell me what the state of the T-cells is, I don't want to know." But someone let it out, in about February, four months before he died.

He managed to go to South Africa for a holiday, he'd been before with my mother which was good for both of them. This time was the January before he died and he came back really topped up – the sunshine helped enormously with the skin, which was really dry and itching. When he booked his flight he asked for a wheelchair.

"Why do you want a wheelchair? What's wrong with you?" "Do I tell them?" he thought, "Do I say I've got leukaemia or something?" In the end he told them he was HIV positive and they told him to ring back in a couple of days to find out whether they'd allow him to fly. I thought that was naughty.

After he came back from South Africa he just gradually got worse and worse. I kept saying to him when he got poorly, is it time you came to me? And he said, "No, I know if I come, I'll lose contact with my London friends." I wanted him to know he was welcome. What began to happen was that he spent more and more time here, the balance changed. Instead of just Friday to Sunday night, it would be Friday to Monday night, then Friday to Wednesday and he'd have to go back for his hospital appointment, and he could go home and pick up his post.

He had a big automatic car so he could drive back and forwards. He was Mr Independent, he'd drive here, come in, fall on the bed and go to sleep. I did worry about him driving, but I tried to think of other things! The car was almost like a lifeline, he loved his car.

He had worked hard in his time and been very careful with his money. He'd got a mortgage but he'd also got some money saved. So he was able to get mobility allowance and things, but he couldn't get the DSS to pay his mortgage because he had more in savings than you were allowed. Yet someone else could get the whole lot paid and that used to annoy him, because he felt his life was going to be just as short as theirs.

Philip and I talked with my brother John about the situation. The important thing is that you do talk to the rest of your family, so you don't feel that one of you is carrying the whole burden, and so that Martin could feel that as a family we were all going the same way and he could feel supported by all of us. Martin wanted to go on living in his flat but by then we all thought he couldn't. But we knew that it had to be him who made the decision, so we had to let him try.

His HIV nurse told him that he wasn't going to be able to cope on his own much longer. One weekend he was here, and when he went back I sent with him a whole lot of bin liners, and said, "Put some of your clothes ready while you're there, while you're well enough to choose what you'd like to bring with you, so that when you do come here, you'll have the things you want with you."

He couldn't even manage that. My brother John went over there and sorted out with him what Martin wanted. Then my husband went down with a van and a large friend and brought back the furniture Martin wanted, and all his clothes. By that time Martin wasn't well enough to drive down here, so Philip drove him back in his car.

We put all the furniture in his room, and unpacked all his clothes. The following week we had to take him back to London because he wanted to go and see the homeopath who'd been very helpful to him at the London Lighthouse. He went back to the flat too to collect some more things he wanted. That was the last time he was there, he was never well enough to go back to the flat.

I went to my GP right at the beginning, and said, "You've seen me through a lot – my little boy dying, my father dying from Alzheimers – now I've got something else. I'm fine – but my brother has AIDS." She was great. She came out and said to him, "Martin I'm going to come out and call on you every Tuesday afternoon, and then I can give you prescriptions and whatever else you need." She worked with the Macmillan nurses and the district nurses, they all came.

So when Martin first arrived we spent two days sorting out who we wanted to help. It all got a little confusing, but it was fantastic to know I wasn't going to be on my own. When the district nurses came to visit, they asked whether I needed incontinence sheets, they brought bag loads of them in, they were really thinking ahead. And they gave me a book which set out where they could turn to for HIV patients – it was really only meant for them but it was really useful. It told you what to do at the death, how when the body's picked up it's put in a bag, and when the undertaker comes you must tell him it's an AIDS patient. I didn't know those things.

My dentist wouldn't take Martin on. I could understand that – and he did put me in touch with a dentist who would. And when Martin went to St George's to have his teeth fixed, the dentist was in a space suit and there was cling film over all the lights! Martin felt those precautions were a little over the top.

When his boyfriend's sister came over to visit him here, in the spring, he was still well enough to go out in the car. We live on a farm and we'd encouraged Martin to buy five bullocks because we felt it gave him an interest down here, and when his friends from London came he used to say, "You must come and see my cows!" So that day he was well enough to get in to the car and shuffle from the car to fence. He wasn't strong enough to walk anywhere, and he fell over a lot. We popped him back in the car, and I drove the girl back to London to catch the plane home, and from that time onwards he just went downhill.

He was still eating. He'd say, "I fancy so and so," and I'd do it, and he'd push it around the plate, although he ate masses of fruit. He'd eat a lot when he felt well, and he was easy to feed, he liked most things.

He had an absolute phobia about smoking in the house, and about the cats – they weren't allowed in the house at all because he was terrified of catching toxoplasmosis. He also used to imagine he saw cats when he didn't, he would say, "Sophie I'm imagining I'm seeing cats". He was well enough to know that he was imagining them, but he was paranoid.

He was very frightened of the illness, particularly about dementia and blindness. I remember once when he was in the John Waring ward at the hospital and there was a man opposite him who was on oxygen all the time Martin was there. And Martin said to me, "he's been like that for ages, the nurses say, he's just hanging on to life by a thread." And that was what he was afraid of, living but with no quality of life. He always said that when the end came he didn't want to be put on any more antibiotics, he didn't feel it would be worth it.

He was very funny about spending money. When his sight got very poor, he didn't go and have his eyes looked at because he said he'd have to buy glasses and spend money and who'd want them after he'd gone! He'd be like that about the car too – a reversing light would go, and he'd say, "Oh no I won't repair that! I'll get a bit of red plastic and stick it on with tape." And then he would feel that he'd saved money – it really made us laugh. He said when he died he wanted a cardboard coffin, we weren't to waste money on wood!

He wasn't a very easy person, he would admit that, and his friends would agree. He never really had a personality change, he just became more difficult. He would lose all his money, he wouldn't know where he'd put his Rolls-Royce book – he adored Rolls-Royces and talked about buying one, so he was odd at times. But we took no notice of it and treated him as normal.

He was very demanding, as if he was the only child, wanting all the attention all the time. If I came home from school, and I was a bit late, it would be "Where've you been? Why isn't my lunch ready? Where's my lunch?" He'd say that in a rather hard way, but he didn't mean it like that.

I'd take Lottie to the ballet in Oxford, and as soon as I came in through the front door it was "Have you had a good time, what was it like, tell me all about it!" It was wonderful that he took so much interest, that helped him a lot. But it was always "Where've you been, what are you doing, why are you doing that?"

I was lucky – my friends were fantastic. My friends included him in everything, if ever there was a party, they all said, you will bring Martin – we don't mind him having a snooze. I had a daily here three mornings a week, and she'd get him anything he wanted. She knew exactly what was wrong with him, and she knew that if he fell on the floor and knocked himself out she was not to touch him but to ring for an ambulance; that if he was sick on the floor, she was to leave it. She knew where to draw the line, and then I didn't have to worry about it. On the days she wasn't here, my neighbour would come in and sit with him. He had a buddy here who would come in every week – she came through Ox-Aids, and I felt supported by that.

I do a lot of work with the hospice and before Martin came to live here I asked them if they would take him at the end, and they said yes. I did say to them, please ask the director and the board – and they came back to me and said, yes we'll have him. They said there was no difference in nursing a terminally ill AIDS patient to a terminally ill cancer or leukaemia patient.

At the beginning he'd manage to get out of bed and get to the loo. Sometimes he'd fall out of bed and we'd be downstairs like a shot. We wondered if we should barricade the bed, but then he wouldn't be able to get out. I did get tired having my sleep interrupted, rather like with a young baby. It was a bit like having another child around the house.

There came a day when I began to have trouble getting him in and out of the bath. I'd been helping him upstairs and bathing him upstairs. I thought, this is no good. I used to be able to sit him on the edge and swing his legs round – he was so slight by then. And he could still help me by sitting on the side of the bath.

But one day I felt it was dangerous. So after that he'd go to the hospice twice a week to have a bath, and they were ever so pleased to see him because he was so full of fun, even at that stage. They had the proper machine there to lower him into the bath and he loved it. He'd talk to them all and they were happy to keep him there till the afternoon, but I knew that he'd had enough by just after lunch so I'd collect him and bring him back home so he could snuggle down in his own bed.

I was still working – and Philip was marvellous. He's self-employed and everyone was incredibly supportive. So he would take Martin to the hospice and then go to work. I'd discussed my job with Martin and told him that I really wanted to keep it on if possible, but I'd give it up if necessary. It's only a classroom assistant, mornings only, but I do thoroughly enjoy doing it!

Having Martin to live here turned our house upside down, and Philip took it all in his stride. Once or twice he'd say to Martin "No!" and Martin would say, "Oh dear I think I've overstepped the mark!" But Philip would look after him, make him a cup of tea, they were friends. We did have one or two rub-a-dub times, when I wondered how I'd cope and was pulling my hair out. It wasn't all sweetness and light.

Martin and I talked about dying – he could talk the hind leg off the donkey. He had a counsellor in London called Luke who helped him hugely with things like when he lost all his sex drive, which worried Martin but it was all part of the disease. He talked to Martin about dying, and Martin talked to us about his funeral. He left me strict instructions that he wanted a very quick crema-tion with just family, and then he'd like a massive party to celebrate his life a month or two later, when everyone had got over his death. Everyone was to come, there was to be plenty of wine.

After he'd been here a month the hospice asked if I'd like Martin to go in for a few days to give me a rest. He went in and I went to Wales for five days – that was a good top-up for me. I felt really mean leaving Martin, it was like leaving him at school. But his friends visited, and everyone there got to know him, the doctors, the nurses.

But when he got back here, I could see a really big deterioration. It had been going on, I suppose, but when you're with someone every day you don't notice it so much. He could no longer stand up on his own, or get out of bed, we had to lift him out and carry him. I had him home for a week and then I was due to do things with the girls, they'd broken up from school. I realised I'd need more help but I didn't know how to get hold of a good nursing agency. I wondered if they would shy off?

It was Martin's social worker who found me an agency locally. They said they'd like to do it – it wasn't so much nursing as being with him, but they said they'd need to know more about the illness. So the social worker arranged for somebody to come and train these nurses, this was in the space of four days. They were taught all about the disease, what they should and shouldn't do, four of them. We arranged a rota, and wrote it down in big writing because Martin's eyesight was getting very poor at this stage. One of them would be here in the morning and give him lunch, and then the next would take over in the afternoon and I'd be back at four.

A couple of days later when I arrived home in the afternoon I realised that he had suddenly deteriorated. His breathing was suddenly worse and I thought pneumonia might be setting in. I rang the Matron at the hospice who said, bring him in, she had a bed. But I told her I couldn't do that straightaway – that would be like saying, right, that's it. I felt we needed time to think it through.

I rang the doctor's surgery and one of the GPs came out. I'd only met this particular doctor briefly before, but he came out and he sat with us for an hour-and-a-half – he ignored all the calls paging him, all mounting up. He told us there were three options. We could keep him at home and have more nursing, we'd need Macmillan nurses and we'd need to sit with him at night. Or we could let him go to the John Waring ward in Oxford, or he could go into the hospice. I asked the doctor what it would mean if he went to the hospital, and he said they'd give him anti-biotics and try and get him better.

I knew Martin wouldn't want to be put on a course of new anti-biotics at this stage. So the hospice was the final decision. I didn't want to rush him off straightaway, I wanted to take him in the following day. I'd like to take my time, get him up, drive him in. The doctor said we could have an ambulance but I thought we'd rather take him in the car.

I was with him that night – even with Philip and I doing it together we couldn't move Martin without hurting him – he would moan, he was in pain. He was very incontinent then, but that didn't bother us – we had all the kit, the pads, disposable sheets. And Philip and I had done the moving for him for a while, we knew how to roll him. But he was moaning.

And I knew he needed something more than my love, he needed a drug. I knew I could have the Macmillan nurses but they don't come out at night and it was at night it seemed worse. Having nursed my little boy I knew that, but he was little, I could pick him up and cuddle him, but I couldn't do that for Martin. I knew I needed some professional help.

Mum was around all this time, but she was distant – she couldn't really cope with losing another child. It wasn't the disease. He and Mum rubbed each other up the wrong way, although they didn't mean to. Mum felt guilty about my having to bear the main burden, but she couldn't have coped, she couldn't have lifted him.

So we got up that Tuesday morning, changed him, got him dressed. I remember I fed him some porridge for breakfast, he always liked that. We put him in the wheelchair and got him into his car – that hurt him a bit I think. But I felt it was nice that we were going to take him to the hospice in his own car. We wheeled him in and he was able to say hello to the nurses. My brother John arrived from London and together we put him into bed.

Matron said we're going to give him some drugs to make him more comfortable, diamorphine I think it was. As we left, Matron said to us, "I can't tell you how long your brother has, because AIDS patients can go on and on and on at the end." That had always been Martin's fear. But he didn't.

He went in on Tuesday morning, and John and I took it in turns to be with him. On Wednesday night it was my turn to go off duty at midnight. I went upstairs, wound up the clock and John came and knocked on the door and said "Martin's just died" – it was ten past midnight.

He died on 30th July, my mother's birthday, and we had a cremation over at Leamington Spa a few days later, and then we had this big party on 3rd September. We sent a note to all his London friends and all the friends he'd made round here – we thought there'd be about thirty. We had ninety people! We had people doing the catering and masses of wine and gin and whisky. The Salvation Army came and brought a minibus full of people – they had been very good to Martin, they run a centre called Oasis for AIDS patients.

We had a service where we had a hymn and then a reading, and then myself and Katie who was fifteen and Lottie who was nine read this poem about hugging. Martin had a thing about being hugged. We read a verse each, and then a line each, and it was very moving – Lottie got the words mixed up but it didn't matter. They really felt they had taken part in the service. The Salvation Army man sang a solo and other people said things about Martin. He wanted it to be cheerful and I think we got that. My mother felt she couldn't cope with it, so she didn't come.

Martin had made a will, he'd listed everything. He'd gone down to Torquay to stay with his solicitor to do this, and in fact he'd become ill while he was down there and I had to go down and fetch him back. I found that to do that for him helped me, I wanted to help him.

He was very organised, he liked to have it just so. He had a book with names and addresses with people to contact. My brother rang me and asked me, "Sophie, would you like me to go over to Martin's flat and get rid of all his clothes?"

I said "Yes please". We all talked to each other, that was very important. And then we went and cleared out the flat, which had been left to me, and we eventually rented it out.

It upset Katie terribly towards the end, not the disease, but seeing him so ill. Katie and Lottie went off to Pony Club camp for a week right at the end of Martin's illness, and Katie was worried about Martin so a friend brought her back from camp one evening. She sat with him, chatting to him. She told him about everything, about the boys in the stables, about the water fights, and about the girls being caught in the boys' dormitory. He couldn't really make any response but she told him the lot. She came away and she was fine and then suddenly she broke down. Lottie knows Uncle Martin died from AIDS, but we didn't dwell on the word too much.

Something which Katie finds hard is at school. They bring in various topics to the humanity syllabus and they have people who come in to talk about AIDS in the community, and she finds it hard. She doesn't open her mouth, not that she doesn't want people to know her uncle died from the disease. But she finds that they come in and talk as if they know all about it and she says, "Mummy they don't know what it's like, they don't know it all."

FRANK is twenty-seven and lives in London with his wife and four year old daughter. He was born in Lusaka, and came to Britain with his parents as a child. His wife was born in Britain to Caribbean parents. His daughter and wife were diagnosed HIV positive when the child was nearly two.

FRANK

When I left school I worked for a year in a bank and then went back to college to do a B-tech, and then got a job with a company where I stayed for two years, until the company went bankrupt, and I was made redundant. I was an inspector of fork lift trucks – I went out to look at machinery which we used to buy and export. I live very close to all my family – my mum is only five minutes away, and my sisters and brothers are all very close too.

I met my wife in 1988, it was very romantic, the usual eye to eye contact. She was a very pretty girl, I thought, let me make a move on her. I met her because my friend was dating her sister, and then we went out together, and two or three days later we were going out as a couple. She was in college at the time, and she was twenty-one. We didn't decide to get married immediately, we continued the relationship for two or three months, and after six months we got engaged.

I lived alone at the time, and she was living with her parents, so she moved in with me. We planned to have children eventually, but it happened that she got pregnant accidentally so we decided to go ahead and get married and keep the baby.

The baby was born in November 1989, a girl. My wife was perfectly healthy at the time. When the baby was about eighteen months, she got ill. She had some swollen glands, and we thought at first it might be mumps. We went to Guy's Hospital, where they checked her tonsils and checked her throat, but they couldn't give us a diagnosis. The glands went down, came back up, went down; we went back and forwards between the GP and the hospital. I did write down some details of the to-ing and fro-ing because I wanted to make a formal complaint about the length of time it took to get a diagnosis.

We really felt the doctors were to blame for not coming up with a diagnosis. We kept on pushing them, and then eventually we said, "Look, we've had enough," and a specialist at Guy's decided to do some blood tests. That's when they told us the diagnosis, after the tests.

They came back and confirmed that the child was HIV positive. It was traumatic: the shock just hit us. Not knowing so much about AIDS and HIV, it not having been part of our family, ever, we had no reason to suspect that was what was wrong. She was a normal kid, she was growing up well until these glands started playing up. And all of a sudden they told us this, and then they suggested that the family as a whole went and got tested. Then they found the mother was positive, though we found that I myself was negative. The shock of finding out that we had this problem which might end up in death was like suddenly knowing your limits. The doctors tried to educate us, like telling us that it didn't mean that the person was going to die tomorrow, but to us it felt as if it was the end. Suddenly we felt like giving up everything – our life was demoralised. We were in tears all the time, and at the same time I had to try and calm my wife down, to assure her that I would still be there. I'm epileptic myself, and I found myself asking myself, "Why me? The epilepsy, my wife, my child both HIV positive, what have I ever done wrong to deserve all this?" We really tried to comfort each other – we had a very strong relationship, and we needed that. We hadn't been married that long, and we were young, we went out a lot, we had a nice life, and now a child as well, but suddenly there was a halt to everything.

I even felt I might want to give up work, but we had to eat, so there wasn't really any alternative. I went on going into work, but I'd ring home all the time to see how they were doing. My wife was in college at the time, and she kept on going in, and my mother and sisters looked after the baby. My family didn't know about this problem. We told nobody at the time and even to date not very many people know. We didn't know how people would react. We weren't even sure how my family would react. When it hit us, we thought, are we going to be treated as second class citizens, are we going to be able to work, what will our friends do. So we kept it secret, just between me and my wife and the doctors. It's always a strain, because you always worry about a slip of the tongue. The worry is about the fact that to be HIV is always associated with promiscuity – that someone will say or think, "Hey, one of you guys must really have been sleeping around." In fact, when we talked it through, my wife explained to me that she had got it from a blood transfusion. She can't be sure, but she's anaemic as well, and there was one time when she was really ill and they had to pump in some blood. It was early 1983, and the blood was not screened. We've been through her ex-boyfriends, and they're all well, some of them have children, none of them show any signs of illness, they all seem fine, so we believe it was caused by that blood transfusion.

I wouldn't have taken it badly, the fact that she got it from somebody else, but it does make me feel better that she got it from a blood transfusion as that clears her name from being a sleep-around. I don't want to tarnish my wife's name, or to have to say

181

that to my family. But if she had got it from another guy, I'd have treated her exactly the same because I accepted her for what she was at the time I married her, and this happened later.

My family was really curious about the baby, why we kept going back to the hospital, and why the glands wouldn't go down. We told the family it was something to do with mumps. In the end the hospital found she had a chest infection, which they said was probably causing the glands to swell up, and they concluded it was TB, as they always do in AIDS related cases. We all had to be screened again for TB, although they didn't find it in any of us. So we told the family it was a chest infection, because they really were worried. My wife was really upset about the baby, we spent a lot of time in tears, hugging each other. I remember the first people I told were my parents-in-law. Her mother is telepathic, and she knew that her daughter was ill. I felt closer to my in-laws than I did to my mum. My parents had been divorced for some time, and my mum was quite a harsh woman, very strict, so we couldn't really confide in her.

I thought she'd say, "Well, why did you marry that girl?" I had that fear, so we decided to leave my mum out of it for the time being. Besides, it seemed right since the problem was really with my wife and child, because I'm negative. I'm only thankful that I will be there and able to be strong for them. So we told her parents. They didn't show it at the time, but I'm sure when they got back to their own home they were shattered. They're very supportive; her mother is a very religious woman, she believes in God a lot. She kept saying, "I never thought this would happen to me, in my family," but she thought it was her duty to support her child. She says "Look child, we're behind you, we pray for you."

Sometimes the baby goes over to my sister for the weekend, and my family gets curious because they have to give her medication regularly. So they began to ask, "What's wrong?" And sometimes I would look miserable, maybe something had gone wrong at work on top of everything else, and they'd ask me, "What's wrong?" So eventually I told my sister. I said to her, "Do you know that I might someday lose my family? My wife and the baby." My sister said, "No, why, what's wrong?" I just told them it was cancer. My mum again kept wanting to know, and again I told her it was cancer, cancer of the uterus, which the mother had passed down to the child. And they bought the story. To date, that's what they know.

I told my brothers the same story. My wife really doesn't want people to know. It's only her parents who know the real truth; we haven't even told her sisters. But the whole family is very supportive, they treat the child in the same way as before: they take her off for weekends, take her out to McDonald's, to the funfair, to birthday parties.

The child is now four, and she goes to playgroup. At the moment she's well: she puts on weight, she plays well, she's an intelligent little person, she asks a lot of questions. She's on a certain amount of medication; she's on Septrin, in a suspension mixture, and she's on AZT. We give her AZT from time to time, but we have reduced it, because there are problems with it. Right now we're discussing with the doctors what medication to change to. Although there was all the publicity about AZT being useless, now the doctors are saying that it does work for a limited period. They recommend switching to DDI or using it in a combination, but again we don't know the side effects of that. DDI isn't used very much, it's still being researched, so we still have to do some consultation.

I always feel she has a chance to make it. I look at my daughter and I think she's been so lucky. You know, they say that by the age of three they get really ill, and she's passed through that stage.

She's a real little fighter. She does have a very nasty cough, very dry, but she comes through it . . . We try to give her a very healthy diet, less sugar, less fat: we are very conscious that she needs the good stuff.

At nursery, we don't worry too much about her catching things. We worry more about other kids catching things from her, if she has a cut or something. The person in charge knows that she is HIV positive and is a special needs child, that she has to have medication, and there may be times when she needs to rest.

She's now registered at St. Mary's, Paddington. Guy's took almost a year to diagnose the problem, and when they did find out what the problem was their attitude changed. They isolated the baby, they put bars round her bed, they locked the door. They said it was because the TB was contagious, so they locked her up in her room. I felt they really began to treat us badly – the nurses were gossiping to each other, and in the end we asked them to find us another specialist. I felt there was real prejudice there which showed after they diagnosed the problem. There wasn't an AIDS unit at Guy's then. But when we came to the Paediatric unit at St. Mary's, the reception was great, even though they told us they were still learning. We felt really welcome. My wife attends the adult clinic, and the support has been excellent.

We know that later on in her life, my daughter might run into difficulties in school. We've been discussing whether when she goes into school we tell them the truth, or whether we tell them it's cancer, or a chest infection, so that they treat her the same as all the other children. She's a very fast learner and she needs the academic education. She might not live long, but she still needs academic development.

Where we live there is a social worker who specialises in people who are HIV positive, and she comes to visit, and she could sound out the school for us in advance, sort of prepare the way.

The child is already asking us questions, although she's wonderful about taking the medicine, you know, she'll wake up in the morning, "Medicine, Mummy! Medicine, Daddy!" The Septrin is fine, but the AZT is horrible; every time she takes it, she shudders. The only flavouring they put in it is apple and she hates it.

We always tell her she has to have the medicine because she's coughing. She gets very cold, and we tell her she needs the medicine to get warm and fit. I suppose as she gets older, we'll start to tell her a bit about it, in a sporadic way.

The only major illness my wife has had was after she had a termination. She got pregnant, and she became really weak – she lost a lot of weight. It was really bad for her, she was really throwing up. After the termination, she improved. She wanted the termination herself as she really worried about the next one being HIV positive. She was really low after that, she cried a lot, she felt she'd killed someone. As much as I wanted another child, I supported her because I thought it was for the best. Maybe as time goes on they'll find a way of protecting the baby, but then we have to realise that the pregnancy will make her ill.

She does get very tired when she's coming up to her monthlies, those are the times when she'll complain of a headache, and feeling dizzy, and she'll rest. She does sleep a lot, and she has been advised to take a rest whenever she feels tired. She doesn't drink very much alcohol, and she was on AZT for a bit. She doesn't believe in it all that much, and when she did take it, it did have side effects: she had really knocking headaches.

Her cell count is pretty low now, and so is the baby's. When the child was first diagnosed she had about 700 T-cells, now it's gone down to 25, which is worrying.

That distressed my wife. She took the baby into the Paediatric Unit for a check-up and that's when they told her this. I rang and asked her how it had gone and she asked me to come home from work and talk to her. Immediately I was worried, I thought, what's happened now? When I got home, she looked so sad.

In fact, I think my wife has got to the stage when she doesn't want to know what her T-count is. I want to know because I want to know what the position is, but she doesn't want to talk about it now.

I don't go to a support group because my wife feels she doesn't want people to know. Sometimes I think I'd quite like to go to a group and find out how other families are coping. The main emotional support we get is from the Social Services at the hospital, and the health visitors who come and visit us at home. And they really do feel for my wife, they sit down together and cry, they're very fond of my wife and the little girl. I think the care we're getting from St Mary's is fantastic, and we certainly didn't get that from Guy's. I come in here and they give me twenty packets of free condoms!

If my wife gets worse, or beyond redemption, I'll tell my family, but it's my wife's wish that they're only told after she has gone. I certainly would tell them what she had died of afterwards.

Once when the baby was actually admitted into hospital, my mum pitched up without warning, found one of the doctors, and tried to get the doctor to tell her exactly what was wrong. But the doctor was very clever and said she'd have to come and ask me.

I'm the eldest in my family, and my sister is engaged, but otherwise my brothers and other sister are all single. I always try and educate them about AIDS and HIV. I always say, "Look, we've learnt so much about AIDS since we've been back and forth into hospital: so do take care, do take precautions, use condoms, when you go on holidays, be careful." They're all at the stage when they're really dating, going out and partying, and that's why I caution them. I'm sure they're all aware of the problem themselves because of the media coverage.

I look at my daughter sometimes, and I think, what next?

The chest infection is still there, with the nasty cough. Some time ago she had a rash, all up her arms and over her front. It seemed to be eczema, but whether it really was eczema or some sort of reaction to the AZT, who knows? We've noticed that since we've stopped the AZT, there isn't so much of the eczema.

We now have a very good GP, but we did have a problem with our original GP, who was a man. He knew about the illness, because Guy's Hospital, without consulting us, sent the results of the HIV test back to the doctor. That's when we noticed that the service we got from the GP changed. The baby would get temperatures, and we would panic, and think, what's wrong? We would ring up the GP, and say, "Look, it's raining, it's cold, could you come over to the house?" And he refused at all times to come over to the house, ever. Once I asked him and he said, "You bring the child over here." This was seven o'clock at night, and we didn't have a telephone at the time, I had to go out to a call box to ring him. The child had a temperature, her breathing was rapid, and she was very hot and sweating a lot. As we had no money for a taxi, Paddington was too far for us to go, and when he refused I said I was going to report him to the authorities, and he just said, "Right, you go ahead."

The next thing was that he removed us from his GP's list – we got a letter saying we had to find another GP. Apparently they are perfectly entitled to do that. We got in touch with the social workers at St. Mary's, and they said they'd do us a letter to a new GP. We found two female doctors, and they accepted us. They've been very good, and my wife feels more comfortable, woman to woman.

I'm still unemployed, but I'm still looking for work. Last week I applied for a position, but I haven't heard anything yet. We're getting the disability allowance for the baby, but my wife was turned down. They felt she didn't need anyone to look after her yet, but we do get income support.

I think the thing that keeps us going is hope, really, and the love and care we have for each other. We keep hoping and praying, and I also hope I can help other families in the same situation. I'm a Catholic and I do go to church. My wife has an inclination towards the Pentecostal church because that's what her mother is. I'm actually thinking of confiding in my parish priest, but I don't know how he'd react. We're getting towards the time when the child is going to be baptised and I wonder is this the time for me to tell him.

My wife doesn't like the idea of the priest coming to visit all the time. When the social workers brought students with them to visit, she used to say she didn't want all these people knowing about her condition. She doesn't want to be dependent on people either, she just wants to be treated normally. She's planning to go back to college to finish her diploma in travel and tourism, so that maybe she can go back to work once the kid is at school.

We want to continue as a normal family for as long as possible, having dinner together, going out to the pictures, driving out to do the shopping, giving the baby the shopping to carry, forgetting about the problems, really trying to be normal.

We take notice of all the news about research into HIV and AIDS, and that gives us some hope.

I think London is an ideal place to be. The social services are there, the transport is good, you can jump on a bus or a tube any time. We have good neighbours who are friendly; we do gardening together, I give them my flowers and they give me theirs.

Last weekend the couple who live opposite came over to tell me all about their problems, they'd been fighting all weekend and were talking about divorce. I found myself acting as an arbitrator, advising one of them to sleep on the couch or in the spare room – at least it took my mind off my own problems for a while.

We've got to the stage now when we're discussing a second child. My daughter is too much with adults now, she needs a child to play with. We've had several options outlined to us; I may have to donate my semen, and do it that way. I used to sleep with my wife without a condom for years, and it makes me wonder how on earth I got through without becoming HIV positive. I'm not going to run that risk now. We might just wait for a while and see what new research and new medicine might come up. I do very much want another child, but I'm not prepared to jeopardise my wife's health. Even now, sometimes she blames me for having this first child, she says, "You're the one who wanted to keep the baby," and we do get into arguments, just like everyone else in normal relationships.

She would really like to have another child; her friends ask her every now and again whether she's planning another one, and then you realise again that you have this problem with secrecy.

We end up telling them we can't afford it at the moment, but I'm sure they wonder why we don't have another.

I think my wife is now very fearful, she often finds the visits of the social workers upsetting, because they remind her of her condition.

She tends to cry a lot; she will lock herself into her room and have a good weep, and I say to her, "Please don't do this." We always used to cry and sob together, but I've just got stronger and stronger, because I know they need someone strong. I need to be strong enough to organise things for them when they get ill. But she says she just wants to have a good cry and get it out of her system, almost as if she enjoys it. I find it's happening too often now, I don't want to see her in that state of distress.

I was listening to a Michael Jackson song the other day at my sisters, and listening to all those words, "Will you be there, like you're my brother." I was enjoying the music and then I found I was having a good cry. But I don't do that often, because I know that this thing will be with me for the rest of my life if they both die. The trauma is not here yet for me, but it's coming, and that's going to be very hard for me to take. They need my strength and support at the moment.

That's why I go on holiday every now and then, on my own, that's a good break.

I get some peace of mind, and I can come back and see new avenues of coping. I know eventually I will have to live without them, and going away on holiday on my own is good practice.

We've had a lot of support from the medical profession, and I feel very much I want to give back to society what I've received. We know that HIV and AIDS has risen drastically over the whole world, and if there's a way I can contribute I will, to support a charity or a trust, to help stop this terrible plague. I've always told my wife that I would start something after she dies, and I'd name it after her.

My message is that people with HIV should not be treated as second class. It's an illness we have to come to terms with, because almost every family will be exposed to it, in one way or another, and if everyone can accept it as a normal illness it will help us to live with it in harmony.

MICHAEL

I'd just done a sixteen-week co-counselling course at the Light-house in London. I'd looked after someone with cancer and I felt that maybe I could help someone with AIDS. Then no sooner had I come through the course than I met a friend I hadn't seen for a while and he told me he had AIDS. I used to visit him and do things for him until he died and I saw first-hand what this illness can do to you. It also made me realise that when you start to look after someone you have to honour the commitments you make to them. You have to make sure you will be there if you said you would be, but you also have to set limits to what you will and won't do.

That came in very useful when I met Charles. He and I had the same theatrical agent, and she took me for tea at his flat. We got on very well and because he knew I'd looked after someone with AIDS he let all the barriers down. He talked openly and positively about having AIDS, never once sounding sorry for himself. We talked about the fact that he'd got some Kaposi's on his face, what that meant to him and how he covered it with make-up. We got on very well, we had lots of interests in common, particularly the theatre.

After that evening I rang him up and said I'd enjoyed meeting him. Although I felt it was too soon to get involved again with another AIDS sufferer, I realised instantly that here was a courageous human being whom I wanted to get to know. If he wanted help and friendship I would be privileged to give it.

I called at his flat the following week in the afternoon. It took Charles some time to get to the door. He was not wearing make-up and looked pale and I thought very tired. He'd been sitting in an armchair with a pillow to rest his head and had been struggling to eat a pot of yoghurt. He'd apparently celebrated his birthday with an Indian meal and had suffered the consequences for several days! We talked for about three hours that afternoon, during which time he began to revive a bit, and began to laugh and tell me stories from his theatre days.

We did make some plans for the future that afternoon. Both of us I think were clear that it would work for us to be in a supportive relationship. I thought I might arrange for him to go to the SAGB (Spiritual Association of Great Britain) in Belgrave Square for healing, and we could have counselling sessions together, and perhaps work on a project. We had a lovely peaceful afternoon together until his energy flagged and I knew it was time for me to leave.

Within two weeks he was ringing me every day and I was doing things for him. In a very short time I was the only one he wanted to deal with and I was taking responsibility for things like his bank accounts. He loved dealing with figures and sorting things out. There's a game I've played with other people, which is quite good, where you say, right: if you were in perfect health and this was your last day, who would you like to spend it with and where would you like to be? And he used to love that because he loved to plan things to do.

I became a structure in his life, and he could depend on me. He had a lot of friends in the theatre who couldn't cope with coming to see him but would send him lavish bouquets of flowers, which he hated. I was always the one dealing with his finances, the rent, the rates, the letters to the DSS, that sort of thing. He didn't want to know about Terrence Higgins, he'd had some bad experience and he didn't want the structure of the Lighthouse. Although he did go there for a couple of visits and enjoyed being waited on – it was like a wonderful hotel and he got spoilt rotten. But he didn't want to know about a lot of the support groups.

I think the main reason he wanted me was that I would always be there, I'd always be consistent, yet I had no history with him.

He didn't really like being with people he'd had a history with and who had known him in a different way. I only knew him as someone with AIDS. He also sometimes got away with murder with me too because as I hadn't known him before I'd put a lot of his bad behaviour down to his having AIDS! I've since learnt from his mother that he was always like that and I let him get away with too much.

I think AIDS patients can get a bit spoilt occasionally. Because there's the terrible stigma about AIDS, they're made to feel very special in places like the Lighthouse, and they get a lot of their own way. It's then very difficult for the rest of us to cope after they've had a spell of "Whatever you want, you're the boss" and all of that.

The development of AIDS has gone hand in hand with the New Age movement and there are a lot of things which have been of great value, the touch, the caring, the love, but that's not for everybody. Sometimes it's quite hard for people to deal with "Everything's all right, you can tell us everything here," and it may be embarrassing to hear some of the open expressions of love.

By the time I met Charles he'd got some Kaposi's and he was very thin. He'd got muscle wastage which I'm sure was from the AZT. He'd obviously been a rather vain young man and he'd obviously been very beautiful, but he didn't seem to suffer from the fact that his looks had gone. In fact he used to get dressed up and walk down the street looking terrible, but in a very loud and flamboyant way. It was a sort of "F... you if you don't like the look of me" attitude. I thought it was wonderful that he could do that. I remember going out with him from the flat one afternoon and making him put trousers on over his shorts, because apart from being skinny his legs were covered in sores. He did look like a leper and I really thought he might get abuse hurled at him.

He'd push me at times to see what I would cope with. Once or twice I'd seen him vomiting the most hideous stuff in front of me and I knew he was testing me to see if I could cope with it. He had a terrible leg, it was all ulcerated, and he wanted it massaging with some oil and again it was a test to see if I could do it. And again I did it thinking, God, this is an open wound, I wonder if I'm putting myself in danger by doing it, and not wearing gloves. Two years after he died I did go and get myself tested because you do start to think, could I have caught it? Maybe one day when I was helping him to bed and I got some fluid on my face or on my hands and my hands were cut?

I never imagined our relationship would go to the extent it did, but I was involved before I knew it. I think that was because he hated different people coming in and out and having to explain things all over again – he said people always wanted to know all the grisly details. He'd stop friends he hadn't seen for ages from coming to see him. He said he didn't want them to see him like he was and he simply didn't want to have to go through the whole thing again.

He'd get wonderful bursts of energy and then he'd collapse. His bursts of energy always involved moving the furniture around, it was an obsession. I moved the furniture around that flat until I thought I'd go barmy! He loved sorting things, he loved organising his bank statements. He wanted his independence, he wanted to hone everything down to the minimum and he wanted to be in control. I think having a goal to work towards is essential and he loved planning the next goal.

I would go into hospital when he wouldn't see anyone else and he'd be in a foul mood but I could always get him to come round if I said, "We've got a bank statement, do you want to check it against the cheque book stubs?" We'd be away, he'd be human.

He decided one day he'd like to make a will, and he was going to leave things to different people. My heart sank at the thought of what that would entail! But then he said, "Shall I just leave it all to you and you can deal with it?" and we thought that would be best. There was no money, but it was like a book here and a chair there. We spent weeks organising that list and then he began to change his mind and say, no, he's not having that chair after all!

I think it's essential to help people to get organised. Some people don't want to talk about death – I'm fine about it, I don't get embarrassed. But organising and planning is so important. And specially that game we'd play: this is your last day and you're in perfect health. Who do you want to be with and where do you want to go? We should all be doing that, shouldn't we? People who are dying sometimes quite like someone to talk to and want to plan what they'd like at the funeral.

I would never have agreed to helping Charles if I'd known in advance what the work would have entailed. But I was very fond of him and it really did feel worthwhile. One of my main emotions was that I was constantly aware of how courageous he was, and it was that admiration that helped to sustain me. And also I always like to complete things, I'm not a giver-upper and I did want to see it through.

I wasn't working very much, so I did have the time to do it. I suppose at times it also felt good for the soul. I could let him take precedence and it was like servant and master, although I had to be firm in how I guided him as well.

He was interesting about sex. Some days he'd talk as if he'd never had sex and it was a mystery about how it had happened, and other days he'd open up and talk about his promiscuity. He hated sex by the time I met him and it used to make him very angry if he saw a sex scene on the telly, he'd switch it off. I was learning as I went along but having done co-counselling I knew it was important to listen, to get him to talk.

I spent a lot of time with him doing all the practical things, mending the vacuum cleaner, doing the washing-up, the shopping. The shopping is so important. People with AIDS need so many prescriptions, so many giros cashing, and the food, the dry cleaning, the washing.

Even now I can pick something up in Marks & Spencer and get that awful feeling I used to get of "No he'll hate it, yes, he'll love it", because everything he loved one day he hated the next. In the food line he only wanted stuff from Marks & Spencer, and things would be wonderful one day and hideous the next and you'd cook it and he wouldn't want it. It's extraordinary that I'm not twice the size really, I ate so many meals I cooked for him and he didn't want!

We did have a lot of funny times. One day he said to me, "You must come and look in this box", and he pulled out the NHS wig they'd given him. It was harder than a brillo pad, made of disgusting dark brown shiny nylon, solid, and he put it on and suddenly it was pantomime dame time! He was very funny about that sort of thing.

I set parameters as to how far I would go – I'd be with him in London but I refused to go away with him. I knew I couldn't cope with that, with the problems of him being ill away from home. Quite apart from being worried sick that he would get ill in some remote place and we'd have to get help, I would have been embarrassed in hotels and places by the state he was in, and he was in a terrible state sometimes.

With what I know now, I would set parameters again in the same situation, with anybody, because otherwise you get worn out. This is as far as I can go and this is as much as I can give. Having said that, with him it was every day. It was an extraordinary year because if I didn't see him one day, we were certainly on the phone several times a day. Sometimes I used to get phone calls in the night and I'd listen for hours to his ramblings.

But he was always careful with me. He could be horrible to people and I don't criticise him for that because what he went through was horrendous. He would be foul to people, especially his mother, but with me he'd always ring and apologise because he knew I could always walk away – his mother couldn't.

We'd spend hours going shopping together – we'd go to an opticians and try on frames all morning, or I'd take him to exhibitions, healers and all sorts of alternative things. I always felt that it was good if he had things planned which could give him a bit of hope. He wasn't a fool – he knew more than the doctors. Often he'd go and ask advice about something and the doctors would admit that he'd studied it more than they had, he'd read more papers. But he did always have a little hope that something might give him a bit more time. He was heavily into vitamin supplements, he spent a fortune on them, but really his stomach couldn't tolerate them.

He was always very open about having AIDS, but I remember one day he was at the hospital being checked out for something and he said, "They think it might be cancer, and that's wonderful

194

because ordinary people get cancer." I realised then that it did bother him, the fact that AIDS had a stigma attached to it. He'd suss people out – if they were simple souls he'd tell them he had cancer because he thought they wouldn't understand or be sympathetic about AIDS.

There were times when I thought he wasn't capable of living on his own any more, and times when I think he thought he wasn't either but he was absolutely determined to. There were times that frightened me. For instance, his skin always seemed to be coming off.

One day I went in to the flat and all his hair had come off. I tried to get it off the sheets and it was all stuck on and he was suddenly bald. I thought then, his skin's coming off, he's going bald, I think this is all too much for me at the moment. He had another friend who came in and did the washing and I'd be glad when she came and I'd say, "Should we get the doctor?" And then he'd put a hat on and go out. I admired his determination hugely. He was just so incredibly brave, he really was, he was such a valiant fighter. As time moves on my admiration for that fighting spirit grows. He was amazing.

He had a thing about euthanasia – he used to make plans to go to Holland and be done away with. Once he got out all the ferry timetables and he was planning for us to go there together! I said, "Hang on, you mean we're going to book two tickets there and one back?" It was so preposterous I remember finding it very funny. In the end I did manage to persuade him that you couldn't just turn up on the doorstep and say, could you please do me today?

About a month before he died he decided to go to America, so he needed a visa. By this time he was incontinent, he could never get up before about noon.

We had to be at the Embassy by about 8.30 a.m., and I got there early in the morning to collect him and he was ready. It was amazing, I don't know how he did it. We got to the Embassy and I got him a sandwich and a cup of coffee. He was being totally incontinent, messing his trousers, yet he managed to get in there and go up to the little booth and sit and talk to the woman who was asking him about the visa. At one stage she mentioned the possibility of him having a medical. I was terrified because I could see his mind working, I thought he would send me in for the medical in his place! But they suddenly discovered they'd been born in the same place and they started talking and she stamped the visa and forgot about the medical! He could charm women, even though he looked appalling and he was incontinent. He could never have passed the medical, but there it was, he had the visa!

There was a classic moment when he was in hospital. I'd visited him every day and he was due to come out the next day. I asked him what he needed me to bring in – there'd always been masses of stuff to bring in every day – and as I was leaving he said, "Oh, and by the way, a dozen bottles of red wine!" He'd just decided to give all the nurses a bottle. So that was another thing, I had to stagger in with all these wretched bottles.

I watched him become a lovely person at times. He wasn't a New Age or slushy person at all but I remember right at the end when he was like a skeleton lying there, he was in a terrible state and he really had nothing going for him, and he just said, "I've really discovered that whatever you lose, there's still love there." From someone who would never have said a thing like that it was wonderful, I was choked. It was such a genuine thing.

A couple of days before he died I went to visit him in hospital and I found a nurse feeding him. As soon as I arrived he stopped her but I was astonished because he'd never ever allowed anyone to feed him. I knew then we were on the way out. He sent the nurse away and asked me to hold his hand. "Give me energy!" he said. "That's so important." I felt there was a great deal of love passing between us and much of it was coming from him.

He asked when his mother was coming to see him, and I told him she'd come any time he wanted and we'd thought Monday would be a good idea. "Good," he said, "that gives me the weekend to rest and have my blood transfusion." Then he handed me his Filofax. In all the time I'd known him, his precious Filofax had been the centre of all our operations. I'd never been allowed to touch it – he'd issued all the orders and instructions from it! So then I took it from him and wrote, "Monday, Mummy."

At that stage he wanted to go to the Mildmay – once he'd had to share a room at the Lighthouse when he'd been there and he

196

thought he'd be better off at the Mildmay! It is a trait that in the AIDS illness the self becomes very important, you're fighting for yourself all the time. He showed me a leaflet then for the Mildmay. "It sounds ideal," he said, "not as frantic as the Lighthouse, proper nursing staff, real peace." He'd finally lost his nerve in the flat, he knew he didn't want to live there any more. "Can you cope with Hackney?" he said with a smile. I assured him that of course I could.

Two days later, on the Sunday, I got a phone call from the hospital to say he'd taken a turn for the worse and they thought I'd better come in immediately. I rang his mother who arranged to come up to London straight away. I rushed outside to grab a taxi – I didn't want to drive in case I felt shaky. When I got to the hospital they were busy – they'd had other people dying that day and could I manage with him on my own? The nurse told me that he'd started to become withdrawn early in the morning.

The doctor did say to me then, "I don't want to do anything heroic, is that all right?" Charles had signed a living will stating that when the end came they were to let him go, and that's what they did in the end. We were very lucky. I was shown into his room. I remember thinking how clean and tidy he looked lying on his back in a neat crisp bed. I sat with him for about three hours.

I held him and talked to him, I'd never held someone while they died before. It was very quiet, very peaceful, the blinds were drawn. I told him to relax, that he was loved, that everything was in order. I was holding him and stroking him. At one stage he gave a loud cough and frightened the life out of me, it was so un-expected in the silence, but the nurse came in and said it was nothing.

I talked to him all the time and if he did start to breathe badly in short gasps as if he was desperate, I really could calm him. We'd talked a few times about whether when you die it's a bit like a tunnel and you move towards a light and I started to refer to that and say, "If there is a light there, why don't you relax and move towards it," and he would relax and breathe better. I could see a pulse beating in his beck, but gradually it grew weaker, and then I became aware that his eyes were opening.

I rang for a nurse who confirmed that he was dead. It was a

wonderful experience to share that, to go through it, rather than someone ringing up and saying he'd gone. His mother arrived five minutes after he'd died. She was so brave, so in control, I thought she was wonderful.

Some time before he'd assured me that I would get on really well with his mother when I stayed with her and I thought at the time, why on earth should I ever go and stay with her when I didn't know her at all well? I realise now that he was setting me up as a surrogate son. And I have got close to her, I admire her enormously for what she went through. I think they are two of the gutsiest people I have ever had the privilege of knowing.

Everyone in the ward was wonderful, there was no lack of love and kindness showered on us. I never felt I needed counselling or anything after Charles died, I felt I'd done a lot of unwinding during the time I spent with him. Three hours is a long time and I think I talked an awful lot out to him then. I knew at times I'd been rotten and there had been times when I'd hated him. I'd kept a diary and a couple of time I'd written that I wished he was dead.

He was incredibly brave. To be dying inch by inch like that and still plan ahead, that was brave. He didn't suffer fools gladly, either – he'd have the nurses in tears sometimes. And no platitudes. You wouldn't dare say, "There, there, it'll be better tomorrow" – phew! He wanted the truth, which you had to mask at times.

That was quite hard for other people to cope with and very hard on families, which is why sometimes if there's a stranger in there, although it's hard to accept, it can be a good thing. I think I coped well because I wasn't really involved on any emotional level and when at times I found him difficult to handle I could treat it like a job. I did what I could as well as I could, but I wasn't like a lover, there was no family feeling, I could be more detached. Though I confess there was many a night I lay awake wondering how I could get out of it.

There were lots of times when he didn't want his mother involved and yet right at the end he refused any more visitors but he did want to see his mother. Some of that was to do with wanting to go back to being a little boy again and to go back to Mum and escape all this, and start again.

Just before he died, when he was still at home, I was in the bedroom changing the sheets, and I was sitting on the bed when he came in and asked what I was doing. I remember saying to him, "I'm just thinking that one day you're really not going to be here, and I'm going to have to clear this flat out!" He enjoyed the humour of that, and of course that day came and I did have to clear the place out.

When it came to his memorial service, I did manage to get everything exactly as he wanted it – the only thing I couldn't manage was that he wanted champagne and smoked salmon for everyone. It would have cost a fortune and I'm afraid he got tea and biscuits.

It took a good three months before I got everything sorted out, the flat, the belongings, the credit cards, the bank accounts, and I think I gradually unwound during that process.

I missed him. There was so much in me that made me wish I'd done it better. I began to remember the times when I'd been a bit short tempered and I had snapped back at him, and I never gave him enough credit for how brave he was. But it did feel worthwhile and in a barmy sort of way I enjoyed it.

I work in the field of advertising and it is extraordinary how high the proportion of gay people was in the industry, and they've vanished. Gays are out – I heard a director say the other day about an actor they thought of using in a soup commercial, "I don't want anyone gay because gay people get AIDS and AIDS doesn't sell soup." I think that most people still think AIDS has a terrible stigma attached, not so much in London perhaps but away from the cities.

When my parents in Leeds knew I was looking after someone with AIDS they were convinced I would breathe in the virus – they wished I wasn't doing it. There's a definite feeling that people with AIDS have brought it on themselves, and yet if we go that far, so is cancer, which can be stress-induced. It makes me sad when people express that prejudice but I also feel strongly that if people carry on having sex without condoms then they are absolute idiots.

SISTER EVA HEYMANN is a Catholic nun who trained as a psychiatric social worker specialising in family therapy. She now co-ordinates the Family Support Network at the Terrence Higgins Trust. Her order, The Society of the Holy Child Jesus, has a convent in the heart of the West End of London. I first met her when I made a feature for Woman's Hour about the fear and prejudice which families who have a relative with HIV AIDS encounter within their own communities. Don't imagine a stark figure clothed in black from head to foot! If you met her in the street you wouldn't know she was a nun, since she wears normal and attractive clothes. We spent several hours working together on this chapter, and I know now why people love going to see her to talk over their problems.

EVA

I've been working with AIDS people for the last five years and I think that there are three main problems which families encounter – there's fear, a feeling of having a stigma and the ignorance in society generally. It's those things which separate out the families with AIDS from the families with cancer and other terminal illnesses.

AIDS is often seen as a modern-day plague because it started in the gay community, and there is still a lot of homophobia about. When I first started working in the field, there was a definite feeling around that although I was not bringing physical infection into the house, I was bringing in some sort of moral infection.

Among the AIDS community it doesn't matter how a person catches the virus but to the community at large that is still difficult. AIDS causes an enormous amount of stress within the family circle because it may not be possible to tell every member of the immediate family that a relative is HIV positive or has AIDS. For instance, the grandmother may have a heart condition and it would be risky to tell her.

Every single family is different but there are some general problems. The first difficulty a person may have once a diagnosis has been confirmed is how they are going to tell their family and friends. Then what follows is the family wonders what it can do to prevent it happening. Perhaps if they have him home and feed him up he will be all right? Or, if we can get him away from "those people", he'll be all right. That kind of rescue operation – the sense that we've got to pull out all the stops and then we'll find the right answer, and anyway there's going to be a cure isn't there? – is a common response to a diagnosis of AIDS.

One of the biggest tensions in families can build up because a sister or brother may know about the AIDS diagnosis before the parents. That's very hard for the parents to take, they may feel very hurt and left out. They may wonder, "What have we done wrong? Obviously he/she thinks we're not good enough, and he/she doesn't trust us." And there's all the past guilt about why they don't trust them, and that can go right back to adolescence and early childhood. It can cause great anger, although the reasons that the person with AIDS has not told them may have been extremely caring – for example, they may have wished to protect elderly parents.

I know one family who managed to stay together until the son died, but have since split up. The parents have separated, the brothers and sisters are in different camps – it was a total disintegration of the family unit. Part of that problem was that there was a lot of anger which was never resolved, and there were a lot of accusations made when the son was ill. The death seemed to reactivate all kinds of unfinished business to do with losses in the family's life. If a family is not together, it can't mourn together.

Then sometimes there's a hostile reaction in the family, "Well, he's brought it on himself and he'd better get on with it, there's nothing we can do." There's less of that than there used to be but it still happens. "He would never listen to me, so it's his own fault."

If a son is gay there's a tendency among fathers to feel very guilty about their son's homosexuality. The unconscious feeling may be "I have not presented the right model." The longer I work in this field the more I feel that you cannot put homosexuality in one watertight compartment and heterosexuality in another, let alone bisexuality which no one wants to know about. I think bisexuality is one of the most controversial skeletons in the cupboard – some married men may have had bisexual experiences in their teens, and maybe again in later life, and similarly some women have a great need for intimate relationships at some stage in their normal maturation.

We need to avoid being judgemental. A real lesson I learned was when I was introduced to a man who had a small son. I had been told the father was HIV positive and I assumed he'd picked up the virus either through promiscuity or through drugs. The story is very different. His wife lost their first child, a still birth, and she herself died from a heart condition. He told me that he became infected because he had a back-street tattoo. His had been a perfectly stable marriage, and neither partner had used drugs. It was a real lesson to me because I had already misjudged that man before I met him. I also thought the child had the virus and I had already "blamed" the mother and father for that.

Parents of gay sons often say at the time of diagnosis, "I always knew he was different but I could never name why." Being different can be felt as rejection, and gay boys often blame their parents and then themselves for feeling rejected. But the difficulty of communication is a fact of life at that stage because the topic of sex can be a real barrier between parents and children. Therapeutically what often appears is a great sadness on the part of the boy that he wasn't accepted when he was young.

Even though the relationship between father and son may be difficult, the relationship between a gay boy and his mother is often extremely close, particularly when the sexual relationship between the parents is not an easy one. There may well be a feeling that as a wife the woman feels diminished but as a mother to a gay son she can feel affirmed.

Families can feel very frightened of being outcast in the community and that feeling is often, sadly, justified. Some time ago I asked an Anglican priest I met what work he was doing among people with HIV or AIDS, and he said "I bury them when nobody else will". It was only a few years ago that a church in central London refused to accept the coffin of a well-known broadcaster who had died of AIDS. Sometimes people are afraid that their jobs will be affected. In one family I know the daughter is the head of a Religious Education department in a large inner-city school. She was terrified that the knowledge her brother had AIDS would mean she might lose her job.

Another factor is the physical threat to people. I know of one instance where someone in a flat in a large inner-city tower block was known to have AIDS. One morning the family went to collect the milk from outside the front door to discover it had been contaminated – someone had peed into it and left a note to that effect.

So living with secrecy is an enormous problem. I can think of another family where the mother decided that no one outside the family circle should know about the illness. And she was terrified of going shopping in case someone asked her questions for which she hadn't rehearsed answers. I have also known family members who feel they can't go out to pubs and clubs for the same reason. So some parents remain absolutely within the family unit and daren't face anyone else. There are very isolated people, and isolation can lead to stress and indeed to a breaking point, which is often the moment at which help is asked for and given.

However, people are beginning to link up and ask each other for help. Even in the more remote parts of the country there are AIDS groups being set up. And many people do phone into London to get information. But many people need time to reorientate themselves from being very disorientated, in order to put up their defences, and you can't face the world until you've got some degree of that.

The feeling of anonymity makes it easy to ring a helpline. A lot of people get help that way initially and then they're put in touch with people like the counsellors at the Terrence Higgins Trust and similar organisations.

It's not always the obvious people in the family structure who will seek help. I know of one Muslim family where having AIDS is a particular stigma because of their religious codes. In this family it's the father who's looking for emotional support and not the mother. She is the one who denies the reality of her daughter's diagnosis, hoping that life will go on as usual and in spite of it. She's also denying her own feelings because her energy is focused on getting on with life. He's the one who comes to the support group. In that case it's a particular problem because it's a girl who's got the virus and in terms of the Muslim faith and similar other cultures that's very poignant for the family and it makes them feel very vulnerable.

Human nature is human nature regardless of being Christian, Jewish, Muslim or whatever. Sadly there are still some people who will not go near anyone with AIDS and will see it as the scum of the earth and the wrath of God. Speaking as a Christian, I've come to recognise the God of compassion who spends His time and gives His love to those marginalised and ostracised by society.

In many communities it's difficult to find appropriate support, particularly when the letter of the law rather than the spirit of the law predominates. I feel we need to widen our horizons and talk not with Muslims, Jews, Christians, but recognise we're talking about human beings who share the same frailties, the same fear, the same sense of guilt, and the same need for acceptance by families, friends, and the wider society in which we live.

Various forms of counselling are readily available. Pre- and post-test counselling at clinics can vary enormously, from five-minutes to an hour, or to three or four subsequent sessions. Counselling also varies depending on how a particular clinic is affiliated to a hospital and to the inter-disciplinary team. Because it isn't always the health adviser who does the counselling it can be different members of the team, and the influence of their own professional training may affect the counselling. There are many centres which offer many types of counselling in the hope of meeting people's individual needs.

The person with AIDS is the person who needs to be empowered, and that's why we do try to talk about "persons" rather than victims, patients, sufferers. When you have a life-threatening disease there is a danger that everyone in your family, including your aunts and uncles and God knows who else, will try to come and make your meals, want to make you cups of tea or invite you out. In other words, to insist on doing things for you. And even with the best of intentions this may disempower you. It also puts you in the stressful situation of having to say "No, thank you, I don't need your help." Knowing that your very condition is hurting people, this is just the kind of attention that will put you in a position where you are more hurt because you're going to have to say no. Nobody likes doing that. So you are involuntarily put in the position of rejecting people. And the process is that everybody out there feels rejected or guilty to some extent about being well when the other person has the HIV virus. That in itself puts a strain on the person with AIDS.

Family members may find it very difficult to see that their way of caring can be a chain round a person's neck. "After all I've done for you – you only had to ask for what you wanted" – how many times have you heard that?

The most important thing a family can do is to be able to grow, and to recognise each other's differences and uniqueness, and the wonder of that. I can think of one family where the girl was very very keen on opera but the family themselves never were, and after her death they became opera fanatics! It began to happen towards the end of her life and she experienced that as them beginning to take an interest in her as a person.

I think we have to grow a great deal to be able to meet each other on the other side, and not to expect people to meet us always on our own ground. There has to be give and take.

It can be very hard for a mother to watch her son struggling to live alone and maintain his independence when her instinct is telling her that he would be better off at home being looked after by her. On the other hand, there is a the generous mother who will say, "His lover has been outstanding, it's totally changed my feelings towards the gay community," and even people saying "I could not have looked after him or put up with his bad temper the way that X did," and that is another side of the picture which I find is beginning to emerge more.

As a parallel I can reflect on the experience of having a series of back operations and I remember saying at one stage to my sister, "I'm not coming home to recuperate until I'm strong enough to cope with my mother's anxieties." That experience taught me a lot, I was constantly having to ward off her need to smother me, which was mutually stressful. But if you don't do that you can become totally taken over and disabled and made to feel the patient, sufferer and victim. I think we have to go all out to enable people to resist that.

One reason for family support is to take the parents off the backs of their sons and daughters and to enable them to be appropriately supported by other people who are going through similar experiences. Families also need to feel held and looked after and it helps to feel they have a forum where they can begin to explore some of the issues about "could we have prevented this?" and what is homosexuality or drug use all about.

Drug use generates another big area of guilt among parents who question what has happened and why their son or daughter drifted away and needed drugs. What many parents find so hard to take on board is that it's not always the lack of providing but over-protection that contributes to the situation. Over-protection such as doing everything for their child from choosing their clothes to choosing friends, who they can bring to the house and who they can't. Sometimes when this happens, and no adequate reason is given, or if it isn't talked through, there's rebellion. If these things are really talked through and the real reasons discussed, children can be very perceptive and are often very ready to co-operate, although they might not always say so. But that's how real principles and good relationships can be built up.

When there's a crisis and members of the family feel they need help that's the time when they're most able to accept help. Like the person with AIDS, the slogan has to be "We empower families to do their own thing". That can be facilitated through so many different ways.

Learning to be kind to yourself is therapeutic, and learning to take responsibility for yourself in order to be kind to yourself is essential. When someone in the family has AIDS there is a need for the rest of the family to look and say, "How are we going to nurture ourselves so that we can all be available to support one another?" And there are many different ways of doing that. Planning a holiday, ensuring that we know what is going to be helpful for each member of the family, talking about it, dreaming dreams and helping each other to realise them, knowing that in this family, where one person has AIDS, everyone is affected. So we all need to learn to help each other.

We need also to learn to listen to what it means to an older or a younger sibling if this relative dies. What does it mean to the next one in line in terms of the responsibility he or she will now feel as the eldest child towards the parents, who may be ageing? We need to allow some of those feelings to come out. In some cases the person with AIDS may have been the child who's kept the marriage together and now that he's likely to die the marriage may break up. So already at that stage the whole family may begin to take sides. That can be extremely stressful for the person with AIDS. On the other hand I know parents who've found that it has taken this particular illness in a child to bring them together, so both things operate.

As in everything one has to find a balance. Both the person with AIDS and the family of that person need support. Both have to find a way of working together to cope with the illness. The person with AIDS needs to feel in control of his life, certainly, but he also needs to go on living in the real world, being aware of other people's problems.

In terms of being the carer, we all have a tendency to want to be the angel of light, to be the "good person". We know within ourselves that we feel very fragile and here we have an opportunity to show how wonderful and generous we really are and as we want to be. It's strange that someone who relies on us, but at the same time may occasionally treat us rather badly, may make us feel quite good.

All of us have a need to be needed. When we're caring for people with AIDS we may sometimes need to stand back and question what motivates us. Who's caring for whom? Am I feeding a particular need I, the carer, may have, by looking after the person with AIDS? We also need to look and see whether there are stresses and strains that may be building up with other family members who are not so involved in the caring. Perhaps I was unpopular in the family, perhaps I was the "baddy", but now here's someone who sees me as the reliable one, the good one, and may be this is giving me, the carer, a much needed boost.

That's why I was so impressed with one boy's sensitive awareness when his parents were staying with him and he was very ill. One night he called his father to sit with him while he was in pain, and he said the next morning, "I usually call my mother, but I didn't want my dad to feel left out."

Initially when counselling I like to meet with the whole family if possible. At that first meeting I try to enable people to talk. It may take two or three meetings to get that process going. I remember one meeting with a family of six members where there

207

were three different cultures in the room. At the initial meeting the person with AIDS said, "Perhaps at the second or third meeting we could talk about death and dying." Very sadly he died before the second meeting. That was a pity because that was a family who could have taken that on board.

Instead what they had to deal with was something that I found excruciatingly painful. Because the person with AIDS didn't want to be overwhelmed by his family's sorrow he had orchestrated some of his death and dying. He didn't have a lover but he asked his friends to be the people who were with him in the room in hospital, and to act as doorkeepers. That was extraordinarily difficult for the family to accept. To their great credit it was the mother who first said "I can understand why he's doing this to us," and they simply sat there, day after day, waiting to be called.

He did call them, and whatever went on between each family member and himself did seem to be healing, but it was very hard on the family to accept that he was in control. For me as the family worker it was also painful to support them in this process. It highlighted for me the need that workers too need support, and fortunately I work for an organisation which recognises that.

The other very poignant lesson that we all have to learn, some sooner, some later, is the value of "being there". We live in a society where we're judged by what we produce, what we do, and AIDS turns that totally upside down, just as true Gospel values turn that upside down. It doesn't matter a scrap whether you've been a producer of a theatre company or a road sweeper, it is who you are not what you do that matters. For the people who are nearest to the person who is dying, being there is important, not trying their own line of intervention, but responding to the needs of the person once the person with AIDS himself knows what those needs are.

The meaning of the phrase "I'm here and the time is now" contains a wisdom I've thought about a lot and I'm trying to apply it and enable family members to do so too. When that happens some of the stresses and strains between family members can be much lessened.

The HIV illness is a very gradual and up and down sort of illness, so there will be times when families will be confused. They may think, especially about a gay person or a drug user, "You're not the person we thought you were. You come from a respectable family, and now that you have AIDS, you're still not conforming to our pattern. You should be ill, letting us minister to you, giving us all a second chance to do for you what we couldn't do in the past, what you wouldn't let us do. And now you have these terrible illnesses, you don't die when we think you're going to die, where we fear you may die, and now you're living again. You may even want to travel or want to enjoy yourself, without us. What about us?"

There can be other tensions between parents and children. I remember a woman of twenty-seven with AIDS who knew she was going to die, and knew her elderly parents were planning a holiday abroad – that was hard. She realised they had a future which was no longer a reality in her life. For older parents what's hardest of all is the knowledge that a son or daughter will not be able to give them grandchildren, that they won't be able to rejoice in his or her career. That of course is true of any child that dies before his parents, and it's especially hard because of the fear and stigma surrounding AIDS.

In any bereavement work, one has to recognise that some of the pain may be to do with past experiences of neglect or deprivation. I spoke to a mother here not so long ago whose son had died and she was not able to grieve for him because she was still thinking about her stillborn child of twenty-five years ago. Nowadays a stillborn child is at least recognised, but in those days she wasn't allowed to hold her child, she wasn't given a photograph of him, she never saw him, and seeing her son die now brought all that back to her.

Adults may find it hard to talk about death and dying but children of three and four years are often very ready to ask about death and bereavement, and need to be given straight answers. I'm thinking now of a grandmother who's looking after a four-year-old whose mother and father have both died. When he asks questions about it she cannot face giving him real answers. She herself is still struggling to come to terms with those deaths, so she talks in terms of "they've gone to Heaven, they've gone away". She avoids the issue and further confuses this very grieving child who may well have quite severe behavioural problems as well as his AIDS problems.

When young adults are diagnosed with HIV/AIDS, it can put a huge strain on grandparents. I'm working with one family where the mother has died, leaving the father and the two-year-old child with HIV. The grandparents had reached the stage where they looked forward to travelling and to enjoying the fruits of their life's work. I remember the grandmother saying to me, "How can I bear to bury my daughter knowing that in a short time I'll have to bury my son-in-law and then my grandson?"

What impresses me about the people in the support groups I work with is their strength. I have met elderly people who are very confused by the news about AIDS which they receive through the media. They sometimes find it hard to fit their relative into any particular category, but they somehow find strength to cope and they are able to talk about their own painful experiences together with others who accept and understand their feelings.

When AIDs affects three generations of a family it's easy then to recognise how much education matters. For example, take a three-year-old who attends nursery school. She is HIV positive. The grandmother who is caring for her because the mother is seriously ill feels very strongly that no one at the nursery should know about the diagnosis. She fears that if other parents know, the little girl won't be invited to birthday parties and nobody will come to her birthday party. These are very real life problems and that's why there is a real urgency about educational programmes.

Another area which needs to be assessed is the needs of adolescents affected by the HIV virus. The very lack of numbers makes it hard to provide support for adolescents. I know of one boy in particular who is highly intelligent, but as his father's illness progressed he dropped out of school. He feared he would be asked questions about his father's appearance, and was afraid that his life would be made a misery by his peers if they found out his father had AIDS. Due partly to cuts in resources supporting children and adolescents, there was no appropriate help available. Eventually, not having socialised with his own age group for two years he didn't go to college and is totally isolated and depressed.

We need to work towards enabling much more awareness

among teachers and school governors and for different policies to be introduced in schools about HIV AIDS. In many schools there are likely to be students in the sixth form or even lower down who are HIV positive. If this particular boy had been in a school where AIDS was talked about openly, he might have felt supported. But in fact he did not dare put up his hand in school during a lesson on AIDS in case he showed he knew too much and I dread to think of the number of children who are in similar situations. There has to be education from primary school onwards about what loving is really about. To have good models of what real loving is in families, in one parent and nuclear families, is the beginning.

On the other hand we cannot think of educating our children in isolation from the rest of the world. When I think of seven-, eight- and nine-year-olds standing by the airports in Brazil to earn a few pennies because they are going to be used to masturbate adults, then it makes no sense merely to talk about teaching love. In that situation authority does have to step in.

Of course in relation to some African and Asian countries problems with AIDS in Britain are relatively small. Whole villages have been wiped out by the AIDS virus in Africa where, if there is nothing whatsoever to do, no money to be earned, no work to do, sexual activity may be the only way to pass the time and express fundamental feelings. We know that in some areas of the world the hospitals can't even begin to administer treatment, the people just lie in the corridors of the hospitals waiting to die. The percentage of people with the HIV virus in the Far East, and among the street children in South America is almost beyond belief, and we haven't even really begun to realise what this is going to be like, or what the implications of this might be for us.

A very effective way of educating children is through drama. There's a very creative theatre company called NETI NETI who have made a video of a play about grief because they have realised that teachers find death and dying very difficult to deal with. A lot more work needs to be done, not through books necessarily, but through things like film and theatre, on the radio and television, and through drama groups. The children's theatre director Anna Scher has done very good work too. We've seen some of her work at some AIDS conferences and it's much more effective than the lectures.

To be open about being affected by AIDS is also a tremendous help in educating people. There is a need to emphasise that no one dies of AIDS, but that people die of AIDS-related illnesses because their immune system is damaged. That in itself can be the first step towards education. AIDS should not be such a horrendous word. We're talking about people whose immune systems have been damaged by this virus, and we're living in an age now when the word virus is very much more acceptable. There are so many viruses it almost becomes part of our everyday life.

I know of one sister who tells everyone that her brother has AIDS because she has to provide an explanation both at work and to her friends as to why she becomes stressed and upset when he's in hospital. She has a family of her own with children at school and is involved in many community activities. She needs her friends for support and in her case, because she is confident in her explanation, most people respond with compassion although of course there are people who are fearful and who retreat from her.

Every now and then I feel there is real hope that attitudes are changing. I sometimes work as part of a group who will go into a parish. We are a team of four or five and this usually includes one person who has the virus. Sometimes we've been able to include a priest who has AIDS in the team. When he tells his story, there is often tremendous shock but invariably in the end it evokes the best which is in humanity. I know one parish where a support system was started, linked in with the local AIDS line, following such a meeting. These meetings also enable families who were previously frightened to own up that AIDS was affecting them, to now say "My son or daughter has HIV AIDS". In many parishes this has been a catalyst to building up the community.

In another area, a dentist three years ago gave up a half day a week for free treatment for people with HIV, and she's still doing it, and someone else said they had a little flat which could be used for families for short holidays.

One elderly lady came to make the tea during one of these meetings. She had no intention of staying but she did and got

212

hooked. At the end, she said "What can I do to help?" And someone said to her "You're good at baking", and out of that has come the idea that since she herself has to make regular hospital visits, she's going to find out if the AIDS ward would like a regular batch of home baking once a week. These are drops in the ocean but they're wonderful. When you see people in the community getting up and doing things, the need to be part of a group is so great that people find themselves joining a "doing" group and it stops them from feeling angry and helpless because they're involved. To facilitate that in parishes is invaluable.

Within the churches I've watched attitudes towards AIDS becoming more liberal. It still happens that priests will not bury the bodies of AIDS people, though less so now than three or four years ago.

We have an inter-faith group and we run a yearly weekend together with Rabbi Lionel Blue, for Jews, Christians and those who have no faith. The theme this year is "Life; is hope wafer thin", and this aims to enable people to tackle the real problems of fear, anger, sexuality, dying and death. People come together and know that they're in a safe environment where they can look at these issues. It is good to know that there are now other similar groups.

In this country AIDS is still seen as belonging mainly in the gay community and it will continue to be regarded as self-induced by a society which will not take responsibility for poverty and unemployment.

AIDS families need to be heard, to be understood, to be accepted. And this really does call for a much deeper understanding of the illness on the part of the community.

I know one young man who was twenty-two-years-old, gay and HIV positive. He received counselling to help him to face his family and tell them the news. He went home and told them and they talked it over that evening. It seemed to go quite well. The next morning he got up and went into the kitchen where his mother was cooking the breakfast.

He said to her "Mum how do you feel about it this morning?" She didn't even look round from the cooker, she just said: "I'm just sorry that twenty-two years ago I didn't have an abortion."

But of course that is not usually the case now. One mother came to see me the other day and she said to me, "I'll always be there for my child" – and being there is the important thing.

USEFUL ADDRESSES

AIDS CARE EDUCATION AND TRAINING (ACET)
P.O. Box 1323
London W5 5TF
Tel. 081-840 7879

AIDS HELPLINE NORTHERN IRELAND
Tel. 0232 326117

BLACK HIV-AIDS NETWORK (BHAN)
111 Devonport Road
London W12 8PB
Tel. 081-749 2828

BODY POSITIVE
51b Philbeach Gardens
London SW5 9EB
Tel. 071-835 1045

THE BRITISH RED CROSS
Beautycare and Cosmetic Camouflage Department
Nation Headquarters
9 Grosvenor Crescent
London SW1X 7EJ
Tel. 071-235 5454

CARA (CARE AND RESOURCES FOR PEOPLE AFFECTED BY
AIDS-HIV)
The Basement
178 Lancaster Road
London W11 1QU
Tel. 071-792 8299

CARDIFF AIDS HELPLINE
P.O. Box 304
Cardiff CF2 4NE
Tel. 0222 223443

COMMUNITY AIDS NETWORK
Chichester
West Sussex
Tel. 0243 538484

CRUSE
Cruse House
126 Sheen Road
Richmond
Surrey TW9 1UR
Tel. 081-332 7227

HAEMOPHILIA SOCIETY
123 Westminster Bridge Road
London SE1 7HR
Tel. 071-928 2020

THE LANDMARK
107 Tulse Hill
London SW2 2QB
Tel. 081-678 6686
(Day centre for people with HIV–AIDS)

LONDON LESBIAN AND GAY SWITCHBOARD
Tel. 071-837 7324

LONDON LIGHTHOUSE
111–117 Lancaster Road
W11 1QT
Tel. 071-792 1200

MAINLINERS
205 Stockwell Road
Brixton
London SW9 9SL
Tel. 071-737 3141
(For anyone affected by drugs and HIV)

MILDMAY MISSION HOSPITAL
Hackney Road
London E2 7NA
Tel. 071-739 2331

NAMES PROJECT UK
797 Christchurch Road
Boscombe
Bournemouth
Dorset BH7 6AQ
Tel. 0202 709510
(The British branch of the US Names Project, which organises a quilt
made from panels with the names of people who have died from AIDS.)

NATIONAL AIDS HELPLINE
(Freephone) Tel. 0800 567123 24 hours

NATIONAL AIDS TRUST
6th Floor, Eileen House
80 Newington Causeway
London SE1 6EF
Tel. 071-972 2845

OXAIDS
Ebor House
5 Blue Boar Street
Oxford OX1 4E2
Tel. 0865 243389

POSITIVE PARTNERS
The Annex, Jan Rebane Centre
12–14 Thornton Street
London SW9 0BL
Tel. 071-738 7333

POSITIVELY IRISH ACTION ON AIDS
St Margaret's House
21 Old Ford Road
London E2 9PL
Tel. 081-983 0192
(Support and information for Irish people affected by HIV–AIDS in the
UK.)

POSITIVELY WOMEN
5 Sebastian Street
London EC1V 0HE
Tel. 071-490 5515

SAMARITANS
Tel. 071-734 2800

SCOTTISH AIDS MONITOR
26 Anderson Place
Edinburgh E6 5NP
Tel. 031-555 4850

SCOTTISH AIDS MONITOR
22 Woodside Terrace
Glasgow G3 7XH
Tel. 041-353 3133

SHARE (SHAKTI HIV–AIDS RESPONSE)
c/o The Landmark (see page 206)
(Support group for South Asian people with HIV.)

SUSSEX AIDS CENTRE
Graham Wilkinson House
P.O. Box 17
Brighton
East Sussex BN2 5NQ
Tel. 0273 608511

THE TERRENCE HIGGINS TRUST
52–54 Grays Inn Road
London WC1X 8JU
Tel. 071-831 0330
HELPLINE Tel. 071-242 1010
LEGAL LINE Tel. 071-405 2381